Failure Modes and Effects Analysis

Building Safety Into Everyday Practice

— GLENN D. KRASKER, MHSA —

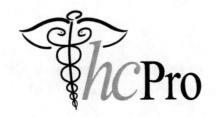

Failure Modes and Effects Analysis: Building Safety Into Everyday Practice, published by HCPro, Inc.

Copyright 2004 HCPro, Inc.

ISBN 1-57839-361-2

HCPro, Inc., provides information resources for the health care industry.

HCPro, Inc., is not affiliated in any way with the Joint Commission on Accreditation of Healthcare Organizations, which owns the JCAHO trademark.

Glenn D. Krasker, MHSA, Author
Ilene G. MacDonald, Managing Editor
Jean St. Pierre, Creative Director
Mike Mirabello, Senior Graphic Artist
Susan Darbyshire, Layout Artist
Tom Philbrook, Cover Designer
Matt Cann, Group Publisher
Suzanne Perney, Publisher

Advice given is general. Readers should consult professional counsel for specific legal, ethical, or clinical questions.

Arrangements can be made for quantity discounts. For more information, contact:

HCPro, Inc.
P.O. Box 1168
Marblehead, MA 01945
Telephone: 800/650-6787 or 781-639-1872
Fax: 781/639-2982
E-mail: *customer_service@hcpro.com*

Visit HCPro at is World Wide Web sites:
www.hcmarketplace.com, www.hcpro.com, **and** *www.healthsafetyinfo.com*

02/2004
18896

Contents

About the Author vi

Foreword vii

Introduction ix

Chapter 1: FMEA Basics 1

    FMEA myths 3

    Why conduct an FMEA? 5

    How to conduct an FMEA 7

    Figure 1.1: FMEA: Preventing Medical Errors from Occurring 11

    Figure 1.2: FMEA Matrix 15

    Figure 1.3: FMEA Risk Priority Number (RPN)—General Guidelines 16

    Figure 1.4: FMEA Action Plan 18

    Figure 1.5: High, Medium, Low-Impact Risk-Reduction Actions 19

    Figure 1.6: Priorities for Risk-Reduction—Performance Improvement Process .. 23

Chapter 1: Related Articles 25

    Examining how workspace affects patient safety 27

    Use FMEAs for more than just regulatory compliance, experts advise 36

Chapter 2: Case study: Blood Transfusion FMEA 39

    Figure 2.1: Blood Transfusion Flowchart 44

    Figure 2.2: Completed FMEA Matrix 53

    Figure 2.3: Blood Transfusion Risk-Reduction Efforts 58

Chapter 2: Related Articles . . . .**.63**

Mistakes and complexity in health care 65

Experts answer questions to help improve your FMEA process 76

Chapter 3: Case Study: Medication Use FMEA **79**

Figure 3.1: Medication Use Flowchart 85

Figure 3.2: Medication use RPN 87

Figure 3.3: Medication Use Risk-Reduction Efforts 91

Chapter 3: Related Articles **95**

Automated system ensures accuracy 97

Medication error report focuses on JCAHO goals 100

Quick fixes won't solve medication system problems 104

Chapter 4: Case study: Patient Suicide FMEA **107**

Figure 4.1: Patient Suicide Flowchart 111

Figure 4.2: Patient Suicide RPN 113

Figure 4.3: Patient Suicide Risk-Reduction Efforts 116

Chapter 5: Case Study: Wrong-Site Surgery FMEA **119**

Figure 5.1: Wrong-Site Surgery Flowchart 124

Figure 5.2: Wrong-Site Surgery RPN 127

Figure 5.3: Wrong-Site Surgery Risk-Reduction Efforts 130

Chapter 5: Related Articles **135**

Projects for improving safety of counts in the OR 137

Chapter 6: Case Study: Delay in Treatment FMEA **143**

Figure 6.1: Delay in Treatment Flowchart 148

Figure 6.2: Delay in Treatment RPN 151

Figure 6.3: Delay in Treatment Risk-Reduction Efforts 155

Chapter 6: Related Articles **159**

Focus on emergency room treatment delays: How stressed is your ED? 161

Glossary of Terms **165**

Related Products from HCPro **171**

About the Author

Glenn D. Krasker, MHSA

Glenn D. Krasker, MHSA, serves as president and chief executive officer of Critical Management Solutions, a consulting firm specializing in medical error risk reduction based in Wilmington, DE. Krasker has worked in the health care industry for 20 years, serving in executive capacities for urban teaching and community hospitals. He also served as director of the hospital accreditation program at the Joint Commission on Accreditation of Healthcare Organizations (JCAHO), where he was instrumental in the design and implementation of the JCAHO's sentinel event policy and protocol. He has successfully coached many organizations through the process of designing safety into their everyday clinical practice, and the challenge of investigating medical errors.

Foreword

How many times have we all heard, "An ounce of prevention is worth a pound of cure"? In health care, the principle of continuous performance improvement has become a mantra for health care leaders. Now along comes this great, effective method for preventing errors by doing Failure Modes and Effects Analyses (FMEA) and we all jump up and cheer—sort of. Doing a root cause analysis on an incident that injured or killed a patient in our own institution is nobody's idea of a good time. Preventing patient injury is a whole lot better. There's just one problem: Who has the time?

Today, health care leaders and managers are more pressured, more frazzled, and less on top of all their responsibilities and challenges than ever before. We are all working as hard and fast as we can just to handle the daily crises we face and fires we have to put out. Proactively making improvements is a great idea, but all too often it's an unrealistic dream given the pressures of the day.

That's where this book can help. The introduction and first chapter provide an excellent synopsis and step-by-step description of the FMEA process. But more important, each ensuing chapter then takes us through this process using an actual FMEA that was conducted in a health care organization much like your own. This book includes examples of flow charts for blood transfusion, site identification, prevention of patient suicide, the medication process, and timely treatment of unstable patients. Each chapter includes a completed prioritization of failure modes for these processes, including their risk prioritization numbers (RPNs). There are also examples of specific process changes designed to reduce the risk of patient injury in these and other key processes. Together, these tools will jump start our own FMEAs, and save us precious time in the process.

Saving time is critical, not only because of our myriad other pressing responsibilities, but also because we have so many high-risk processes to address. The Joint Commission on Accreditation of Healthcare Organizations (JCAHO) now requires all accredited hospitals to carry out at least one FMEA each year on a high-risk process. At the pace of one per year, how long will it take to work through all the high-risk processes in our organizations? Forever! In fact, other high-risk industries perform FMEAs on a frequent and regular basis.

Eventually in hospitals and other health care organizations, we'll all be doing 10, 20, or even 30 FMEAs per year. As a start, if we are going to perform even a fraction of that many FMEAs in our organizations, we'll definitely benefit from the jump start Mr. Krasker provides throughout these pages.

Remember, we're not performing FMEAs simply to fulfill a JCAHO requirement. The goal of every FMEA, in fact the goal of all our improvement activities, is to provide better, safer care to our patients who entrust their care to us. It's the least we owe them to earn that trust anew every day.

Richard Sheff, MD *chairman and executive director*
The Greeley Company, a division of HCPro, Inc.

Introduction

What is an FMEA?

Murphy's Law states that "If anything can go wrong, it will." Thanks to this reality of life, we must anticipate what can go wrong and prevent it from doing so. Simply put, a Failure Modes and Effects Analysis (FMEA) is a powerful, systematic, and analytic tool that is used to identify *where* people, equipment, supplies, information, systems, and processes can "go wrong" or malfunction (potential failure modes)—and prevent them from doing so. If it is impossible to totally prevent such a malfunction, then we can use FMEAs to reduce the impact (effect) of the malfunction on the process, system, person, or other ultimate outcome.

To prevent errors, organizations use FMEAs, which identify the causes of failures or how "things go wrong." They lead an FMEA team through the process of redesigning these flaws so that they do not recur. In essence, FMEAs reduce risk in the process, system, and ultimately the organization.

An FMEA is also known as a Failure Mode and Effects Criticality Analysis or a prospective Root Cause Analysis.

An FMEA can also be thought of as a brainstorming and prioritization risk assessment process that ultimately identifies actions that help reduce risk in and to an organization. The ultimate goal of an FMEA is to ensure that an organization identifies and addresses the most critical failure modes of a system, process, piece of equipment, supply, or flow of information before they occur. It is an anticipatory process that reduces the risk of harm, cost, and exposure to an organization. It is an assembly of group activities provided through documentation of potential failure modes of equipment or processes and its effect on the performance of the equipment or process. Teams composed of various areas, departments, and disciplines will be responsible for performing FMEAs.

Historical background

Although relatively new to the health care industry, the roots of FMEAs go back to the 1940s and 1950s when the aerospace industry and U.S. military introduced the concept. Reliability engineers first used FMEAs as an evaluation technique to determine the effect of system and equipment failures. They classified failures according to the impact on mission success and personnel/equipment safety.

The U.S. military requires FMEAs for all systems to ensure safety as well as reliability. And, for the most part, FMEA has become an indispensable tool for the aerospace industry. Although there are several types of FMEAs (such as system, process, product, design, and materials) and approaches, one common factor has remained through the years—resolving potential problems or risks before they occur.

For years, FMEA has been an integral part of product development in major industries. It has evolved into one of the most powerful and practical process control, reliability, and risk assessment tools for manufacturing environments. Most notably, the automotive industry has adopted FMEAs to evaluate risk in automobile design and manufacturing. The American Society for Quality and the automotive industry have standardized FMEA reference manuals, procedures, reporting formats, and technical nomenclature for that industry.

What we've learned from other industries

Stories from the airline industry abound with examples or how FMEAs benefit everyday safety. Although airline travel is considered to be one of the safest modes of transportation, there is ample opportunity to reduce the risks associated with the industry's complex mechanical systems, physics, and communications.

Statistics reveal that in the United States alone, one emergency evacuation occurs on average every 11 days. Escape slides display a 37% failure rate. The combination of these two factors clearly illustrates the opportunity to reduce the risks associated with airline travel.

For example, although airlines routinely test their emergency lighting systems, during one accident passengers could not see the emergency lights through the thick smoke, even though the battery was fully charged. In another accident, the emergency light went out after two seconds. As the saying goes, the best laid plans . . . .

When conducting an FMEA, it will be clear that some aspects of an organization's operation are beyond one's immediate control. Going back to the airline example, we can expect approximately 10% of passengers to exhibit some form of panic behavior during an emergency evacuation situation. Airline officials might ask, "What can we do prevent such reaction or behavior?" Given the difficulties of controlling human behavior, a more appropriate question would be, "What can we do to minimize the *effect* of such behavior on the overall safety of our passengers and crew?"

Consider the following statistics: 44% of passengers report that they neither listened to the pre-flight safety briefing nor read the safety card that explains how to get out of the aircraft. Fifty percent of passengers involved in emergency evacuations report leaving the aircraft with carry-on bags. These statistics reveal why it's important to identify as many potential problems as possible, anticipate their occurrence, and plan accordingly to reduce risk.

Given that similar stories from the health care industry abound, there exist many opportunities to learn from other industries and to proactively reduce the risk within our organizations. This book will explain how to conduct an FMEA and ultimately to make our organizations safer.

How this book is organized

Chapter 1 will describe the essentials of FMEA, including the following points:

- Why it is important to perform FMEAs
- How to conduct an FMEA
- The step-by-step process
- Prioritizing your highest risk areas

The remaining chapters, 2 through 6, will present case studies that illustrate and bring to life the instruction in Chapter 1. The five case studies include FMEAs on

- blood transfusions
- medication use
- patient suicide
- wrong-site surgery
- delay in treatment

Along the way, there will be useful graphs, flowcharts, and other FMEA tools.

As we start our study of FMEAs, keep in mind that an FMEA is a process or methodology for documenting identified risks and potential actions to improve the safety of a process, piece of equipment, or system. As with any other performance improvement tool, an FMEA is not a problem-solver. It is used in combination with other problem-solving tools, and, as such, the FMEA presents the opportunity to solve the problem. However, conducting an FMEA in itself does not solve the problem. Designing and carrying out risk-reduction strategies is what actually solves the problem, or at least reduces the risk that a problem will occur. As participants in this risk-reduction effort, the latter challenge is up to us.

Chapter 1

FMEA Basics

CHAPTER 1

FMEA Basics

As suggested in the Introduction, Failure Modes and Effects Analysis (FMEA) is an easy to use and yet powerful, proactive engineering tool that helps to identify and counter weak points in systems, processes, and equipment. The structured approach makes it easy to follow, even for those who have not participated in an FMEA before. The benefits that groups and organizations reap from conducting an FMEA greatly outweigh the investment in time, thought, and energy that is necessary to complete, such an analysis.

FMEA myths

Before we get into the heart of conducting an FMEA, it might be helpful to dispel the following myths about this powerful tool:

Myth: *Those unfamiliar with the process that the organization is studying can conduct FMEAs.*

Fact: Contrary to popular belief, FMEAs can't be performed in a vacuum. As we will learn in this chapter, individuals who are closest to and actually carry out the processes the organization plans to study need to be involved in a FMEA. Since these individuals are most familiar with the nuances of the process, their perspectives and input are vital to the success of an FMEA.

Myth: *An individual can conduct an FMEA.*

Fact: By its very nature, an FMEA is a group exercise. It is a highly interactive process that relies upon reaching consensus among a variety of perspectives and opinions.

Myth: *An organization should conduct FMEAs to satisfy a third-party requirement, such as the Joint Commission on Accreditation of Healthcare Organizations (JCAHO) and not to improve a process.*

Fact: An FMEA is a process used to reduce the level of risk to an organization's patients, visitors, staff, and assets. Although they are a means toward complying with the JCAHO standards, FMEAs are solid management tools that should be part of every well-functioning organization.

Myth: *Once the team identifies its risk priorities, an FMEA is complete.*

Fact: While there is a natural inclination to pat oneself on the back and claim the process "fixed" after completing an FMEA, the sign of an effective FMEA is what one does with the information following its completion. As we will learn in this chapter, the result of a well-done FMEA should be a solid plan with actions, accountabilities, timelines for implementation, and measures of success all clearly specified. An FMEA is a dynamic tool that needs to be reviewed and revised during the life of the system or process.

Myth: *An FMEA is too complicated/too time consuming.*

Fact: Although FMEAs do take considerable thought, time, and energy, their benefits clearly outweigh the investment. This book will help guide organizations through an FMEA step-by-step so that they will be able to conduct FMEAs in an efficient manner and stay on track with their improvements.

Why conduct an FMEA?

There are obvious and not-so-obvious clues that an FMEA might be in order. Consider the following:

- *Organizational data indicates the facility needs to proactively reduce the risk of medical error.* A routine and ongoing review of incident reports and trends may clearly indicate that the organization has some systems or processes that place patients at risk for harm.

- *The experience of other, similar organizations and outside literature.* During conversations with colleagues, or while reading the news, health care trade publications, or journals (such as the New England Journal of Medicine), it becomes obvious that other facilities are having difficulty keeping patients safe from certain risks within their organizations.

- A *review of the JCAHO Sentinel Event database reflects that there are known risks in certain systems or processes within hospitals.* The JCAHO Sentinel Event Database provides a wealth of useful information about the types and incidence of sentinel events (those systems and processes known to have caused harm to patients). The elements of performance for JCAHO standard PI.3.20 requires that when an organization selects a high-risk process to analyze, it should base the choice, in part, on information the JCAHO publishes periodically about the most frequent sentinel events and risks.

- *The data suggests it.* There are many sources of medical error incident data and threats to patient safety, such as the U.S. Pharmacopoeia's two medication error reporting programs— MEDMARX℠ and the Medication Errors Reporting program. Also, ECRI (formerly known as the Emergency Care Research Institute) is a nonprofit health services research agency that provides publications, information, and consulting services for health care technology assessment, risk and environmental management, and patient safety. The JCAHO tends to hold ECRI recommendations and position statements in high regard when it comes to improving the safety of patient care equipment and the environment. Based upon information published by these sources, organizations should look at what's occurring (or not occurring) in their facilities to determine whether they need to conduct an FMEA in a specific area or on a given topic.

- *Following a string of related near-misses, an organization realizes it needs to quickly act to avert a true catastrophe.* We must be aware of what's going on within our organizations. The "grapevine" is one of the most valuable sources of information regarding the need to conduct an FMEA. It is well known that medical errors and "near-misses" are significantly underreported. Our own incident reports may not identify that our organization has experienced five nearly fatal medication errors with six months. Subsequently, our leaders would not be aware of the risk that exists within the facility. Confirming the rumors that abound in an organization can quickly lead to identifying trends worthy of an FMEA.

- A *sixth sense tells an organization that something isn't right with a process.* We all know the insecure feeling, deep in the pit of our stomachs, that a process has a greater than average chance of failing. When in doubt, perform an FMEA on the process or system that just doesn't feel right. Similarly, canvass staff and ask them which system or process concerns them the most relative to the risk of failure (where in the organization do they think the next medical error or near-miss will occur).

- A *desire to stay off the front page of the news.* We've all read the horror stories about medical mistakes that could have been prevented. A well-designed and well-executed FMEA in the right area of focus can easily help prevent an organization from being the day's top story.

- *The* JCAHO *says so.* If organizations still need a convincing argument as to why they should conduct an FMEA, the JCAHO requires that organizations select a high-risk process to analyze each year. The FMEA is one way to comply with this standard. Specifically, standard PI.3.20 in the JCAHO's 2004 *Comprehensive Accreditation Manual for Hospitals* (CAMH) requires hospitals to "proactively seek to identify and reduce risks to the safety of patients." The following elements of performance listed under this standard require that the organization:

  - "Selects a high-risk process to analyze (at least one high-risk process is chosen annually)
  - Identifies the ways the process could break down or fail (failure modes)

- Identifies the possible effects that a breakdown or failure could have on patients and the seriousness of those possible effects (*the effects*)
- Prioritizes the potential process breakdowns or failures
- Determines why the prioritized failures could occur
- Redesigns the process/underlying systems to minimize the risk of the effects on patients
- Tests and implements the redesigned process
- Monitors the effectiveness of the redesigned process"

In addition to the above reasons as to *why* an organization should conduct an FMEA, they may also suggest *where* in the organization (which system or process) is an appropriate subject of an FMEA.

How to conduct an FMEA

Having gained an appreciation for some of the reasons that an organization would have to carry out an FMEA, we can now turn our attention to the essentials and logistics of actually conducting one. There are 10 essential steps to this process.

1. Select (using the suggestions in the preceding section) the **system** in which to reduce risk. Consider these questions: Does the organization have lingering concerns over its medication use or the blood transfusion system? Does incident report data point toward the need to reduce the risk of an organization's surgical system?

2. Select the **process** in which to reduce risk. Once an organization narrows in on a system that should be the focus of an FMEA, select the process that has been shown to be the most problem-prone. Processes that are very complicated and have many highly interrelated steps are good candidates for an FMEA. Likewise, processes that are heavily dependent upon human intervention or are not regimented (nonstandardized) are also good candidates for an FMEA. Processes that involve multiple handoffs—especially among staff of different departments—are particularly problem-prone, as are those that

occur under intense (or conversely, loose) time constraints. When staff members have to rush to do an activity or sit for long lengths of time between steps, they are at a higher-than-usual risk for committing an error.

When an organization selects a high-risk process, it mustn't become overly ambitious by expecting that it can improve an entire system (such as the medication use system) at once. The team that conducts the FMEA shouldn't bite off more than it can chew by attempting to reduce the risk of medication ordering/prescribing, transcribing, preparing, dispensing, and administrating processes all at once. Narrow the focus to the process that is the most problem-prone or has generated the greatest concern in the organization. This initial step will take some prioritization, but will be well worth the time. Those that fail to take this step, will find the FMEA process frustrating because it's impossible to fix everything at once.

3. **Organize** the team. Once an organization identifies the process to subject to an FMEA (the leaders of the organization should play a significant role in making this determination), it is time to organize the team. Start by identifying the right participants. Seek out a member of the organization who has education or experience with FMEAs (such as a risk manager who has attended a seminar on how to conduct an FMEA). As mentioned earlier in this chapter, the team should certainly include the individuals who are closest to and actually carry out the processes to be studied. As these individuals are most familiar with the nuances of the processes, their perspective and input is vital to the success of an FMEA. The interdisciplinary team will most likely have representatives from the departments or areas that have the largest involvement in the process under review.

An important factor to keep in mind when pulling together staff from disparate departments of the organization is that many of them come from very different clinical and professional backgrounds, each with a limited knowledge of the other departments' roles in the process. Nurses from the operating room understandably are not familiar with what technologists do in the laboratory, and vice versa. Staff from different health care departments don't always speak the same language—so reserve time in the FMEA meetings to allow staff from the various disciplines and departments to orient one another to what jobs they perform.

Likewise, critical to the success of an FMEA is a good facilitator—someone who is knowledgeable of and well versed in the process of conducting an FMEA. The facilitator should also be a leader who is nonjudgmental, encourages all of the team members to participate and share their insight, all the while keeping the discussion going.

When conducting an FMEA, organize a core team that is consistently involved in conducting the entire FMEA and ad-hoc groups of participants. These ad-hoc groups are invited to join select meetings of the FMEA team when the discussion is going to explore their area of expertise and center on facets of the process with which the groups are most familiar. This approach could be taken to the next level by creating a small team that participates in all the organization's FMEAs. This group will develop a high level of expertise in the FMEA process and can draw on the subject matter expertise of other members who are familiar with the process under analysis.

Once the team is assembled, a good kick-off meeting consists of orienting the team members to their charge (what they are being held accountable for accomplishing) and what is expected of them (first and foremost, consistent attendance at the FMEA sessions, active participation, and contributing knowledge expertise). The team leader or facilitator should develop a common baseline of understanding among the team members relative to what an FMEA is and how to conduct one. Thus, basic education on the essential elements and logistics of an FMEA would be most appropriate at this first meeting.

There are differences of opinion as to whether management should direct and select the representative(s) from each area or department to serve as members of the FMEA team or whether the organization should seek volunteers. As this is an organization-specific decision, it is best left up to the organization's leaders. This seemingly minor decision is in reality extremely important, however, because the choice made by the organization communicates an important message either way. If volunteers are sought, the organization is saying it is seeking those members of the staff with enough passion and commitment to want to improve processes. This will ensure a high level of commitment from team members and will eventually differentiate such individuals from those who don't volunteer. It may also lead to criteria for reward and recognition for those who do volunteer. Among the minor drawbacks of this approach is that the most qualified individuals may not participate in the FMEA.

If everyone is expected to participate in an FMEA at some time and the organization selects the team members, it is communicating that every member of the staff (not just a select few) is expected to contribute to improving processes. The disadvantage to this approach is that it will place individuals who do not have a high motivation for driving change in important roles in FMEA teams, and the overall performance of the FMEA team may suffer as a result.

Senior leadership should be visible to the team members at regular intervals throughout the FMEA process so that the members understand and are reminded of the importance of their team's activities and results.

Other than the FMEA team membership, follow the basic rules of meetings—provide advance notices, maintain meeting minutes or records, establish the meeting ground rules, provide and follow an agenda, and do not allow interruptions. In order to keep up the attendance and participation, agree on a regular (weekly) day of the week and time of day for the FMEA meetings and distribute this schedule immediately following the conclusion of the first meeting. Lastly, the facilitator should manage time well by keeping the discussion and progress on track and reaching consensus among the participants.

Once the team is in place, it's time to get started. A step-by-step process of an FMEA would look like the following:

Figure 1.1 ■■■ **FMEA: Preventing Medical Errors from Occurring** ■■■

- Identify the steps in the process where there is, or may be, undesirable variation (failure modes) by flow-charting the process and analyzing the way the process is actually (and intended by policy and procedure to be) carried out.

- For each identified failure mode, identify the possible effects on patients (the effect), and how serious the possible effect on the patient could be (the criticality of the effect).

- For the most critical effects (based on prioritization), conduct a root cause analysis to determine why the failure mode leading to that effect may occur.

- Redesign the process/underlying systems to minimize the risk of that failure mode or protect patients from the effects of that failure mode.

- Test and implement the redesigned process.

- Identify and implement measures of the effectiveness of the redesigned process.

- Implement a strategy for maintaining the effectiveness of the redesigned process over time.

---

4. **Flowchart** the process. Create a pictorial flow of the process using generally recognized flowcharting principles. Be detailed, but don't get too caught up in perfecting the flowchart. As with any flowchart, focus on the individual tasks that occur and the sequence in which they occur. Flip charts or dry erase boards are invaluable tools when conducting this group exercise of drawing the flowchart.

Start by sketching out the major steps in the process and then have the team members add in greater amounts of detail, based upon their specific knowledge of how the process works in the organization. A word of caution when conducting this exercise: Make sure the team flowcharts the process as it actually occurs in the organization and not as the members want it to occur, wish that it occurred, or how other organizations do it. The key is to focus on how the organization carries out the process so that the team can improve it—so be sure to start with reality.

During (or immediately after) the flowcharting process, have a team member record the flowchart in a computer software package designed for flowcharting. This software provides the capability of sending the flowchart to all team members in advance of the next meeting for their review. In addition, the team can easily change the document before it is finalized. As the flowchart is the foundation of the entire FMEA, don't rush it—allow sufficient time to identify all of the steps in the process. The flowcharting of the given process is usually enough to fill a single meeting's agenda.

5. Identify **potential failure modes.** Once there is general agreement (the term "general" is stressed here because a group rarely can achieve total agreement on the flowchart of the process), ask team members to identify where the process can break down or where failure or errors can occur. Ask the following questions:

   • Which steps in the process (the connectors in the flowchart) can fail?
   • How can they fail?

A brainstorming technique lends itself well to this step in the FMEA. This exercise allows participants to suggest potential failure modes off the top of their heads. FMEA team members speak up and suggest ways in which the process under study can fail. A facilitator records the suggested failure modes and then the group works to reach consensus on a final list of failure modes.

Drawing the flowchart on a dry erase board is one useful strategy for identifying potential failure modes. As you review each step and ask the team how that step can fail in general, or has failed in the organization, bullet each potential failure right on the flowchart—directly under the step in the process to which the failure mode applies. (With the right flowcharting software and an LCD projector, this same method can be projected onto a screen and the ideas saved on the computer at the same time.)

Front line staff who carry out the particular process every day must participate in the discussion. These individuals know what can go wrong and how the process has broken down in the past. Likewise, involve staff who can look at the process with a more objective eye and articulate theoretically how the process can go awry (managers work well in this situation).

6. Identify the potential **effect** of each failure mode on the patient and the criticality of the effect (how serious the possible effect can be on the patient). This unique step is what makes an FMEA a true FMEA. For example, in the medication ordering process, a prescriber's illegible handwriting (the failure mode) can easily lead to the wrong drug being dispensed and administered (the effect).

The criticality of each failure mode helps prioritize which failure mode the organization will attack (or reduce the risk of) first (recalling that it's impossible to fix everything at once). Identify the potential failure modes by determining the following factors:

- *Frequency* (how likely it is for the failure to occur)
- *Severity* (how serious the impact of this failure is on the patient)
- *Detectability* (how easily the failure is recognized or discovered)

Using a 10-point scale, have the FMEA team reach consensus on each of these three factors for each of the potential failure modes. Accomplish this exercise either by having each member voice his or her expert opinion and averaging the responses (a form of multivoting) or having an individual volunteer or call out what he or she thinks the frequency of the failure mode is and allowing the group to reach consensus on a final decision. Thus, for each potential failure mode, the group will agree upon three numbers, each between one and 10 (the frequency, severity, and detectability).

The key to success at this stage is for the team to be consistent in its assigning a number to each factor for each potential failure. The facilitator needs to regularly conduct a reality check to make sure the team isn't assigning numbers that are out of proportion. Checking for face validity—or whether the result appears reasonable and will work—often helps to make sure that the assigned numbers make sense when individuals step back and look at them all.

The rationale for quantifying these three factors for each potential failure mode is that failures need to be weighted according to seriousness. Since the three factors all carry a fairly equal weight in terms of their impact on the ultimate outcome of a situation, they are treated as equal for the sake of an FMEA. If a given failure that doesn't greatly affect the patient's overall care (the severity) were to occur with albeit a high level of frequency, an organization probably wouldn't place that failure high up on its list of priorities of processes to fix first. On the other hand, if a failure was deemed to place patients at considerable risk and it occurred with relative frequency, then it probably would get much needed attention sooner rather than later.

The success of this step in the process is dependent upon the skills of the facilitator. A good facilitator will allow the team's discussion to free-flow without

- letting one member (or a few members) dominate the decision-making or overly influence others' opinions
- allowing the discussion to drag on until members surrender to a decision out of the sheer exhaustion of a protracted debate

This step in the FMEA can be challenging as the team works to reach consensus on the assigned numbers.

For each failure mode, list the frequency, severity, and detectability in a matrix similar to the one that appears in Figure 1.2 and then multiply the three numbers to define the risk priority number (RPN). The RPN equals the frequency times the severity times the detectability.

Figure 1.2 — **FMEA Matrix**

Potential failure mode	Potential effect of failure mode	Frequency (likeliness scale) 1–10	Severity (potential for harm) 1–10	Detectability (potential discovery) 1–10	Risk priority number (RPN)
Identify potential failures for each step in the process	Identify potential outcome of failure to patient	On a scale of 1–10 (10 = highly likely), identify the likelihood of this failure actually occurring Example: 1 = Remote probability 5 = Moderate probability 10 = Very high probability	On a scale of 1–10 (10 = worst potential failure outcome), identify the potential severity of the consequences of this failure Example: 1 = Very minor outcome 5 = Moderate outcome 10 = Very severe outcome	On a scale of 1–10 (1 = failure easily discovered under normal circumstances is highly likely), identify the potential difficulty of discovery of failure Example: 1 = Certain detection 5 = Possible detection 10 = Cannot detect	RPN = Frequency X Severity X Detectability

Given the math, the RPNs could range from 1 to 1,000. As a general rule of thumb, using the table in Figure 1.3, an organization's efforts to reduce risk will focus on those failure modes with an RPN of greater than or equal to 250. However, this threshold may be different in organizations that tend to score RPNs consistently high or consistently low. Again, the most important factor in comparing RPNs is consistency within the organization in how the scoring scales are applied.

| Figure 1.3 | FMEA Risk Priority Number (RPN)–General Guidelines |

RPN score	Relative importance
≥ 250	Significant
100–249	Less important
< 100	Not important

For the most critical effects (those with RPNs of ≥ 250) determine why the failure mode may occur. This will be the foundation for the development of the organization's action plan to reduce risk.

7. **Redesign** the processes/underlying systems. The next step in the FMEA is to identify risk-reduction strategies for the highest-ranking failure modes. The team should brainstorm actions that the organization could take to possibly reduce the risk (reduce the severity and likelihood of occurrence [frequency] while increasing the detectability) of a failure. This brainstorming exercise requires the input of staff members who work closest with the process, as they can best identify how to improve the safety of their everyday activity for the patient.

It is also expected at this point that the FMEA team will find out how other organizations have reduced their risk of the process under study. Speak with, visit, and request policies and procedures from similar organizations to learn how they perform the process safely. As part of this national and local benchmarking effort, conduct a literature search on the practice of other organizations.

At this stage of the FMEA, the team is starting to redesign the process (more specifically the steps in the process and how they work together) to minimize the risk of individual failure modes and to protect the patient from the effects of the failure. Next, conduct an assessment of each potential improvement to determine the extent to which the proposed risk-reduction effort will actually work and what potential impact the change will have on the remainder of the process. Ask yourself, "will this change [risk-reduction effort/improvement] at Point A in the process have an unanticipated impact at another point?" If so, this factor needs to be taken into account before implementing such a change. The underlying question for each change under consideration should be how effective will it be in reducing the likelihood that the process as a whole will fail. The goal of the FMEA team should be to carry out changes at the highest priority failure modes that are most powerful in reducing the risk of failure in that process.

As the team identifies risk-reduction strategies, the facilitator should assign an individual to take the lead in carrying out the effort and organize the results into a matrix similar to that in Figure 1.4.

Figure 1.4 **FMEA Action Plan**

Potential failure mode	Responsible party	Risk priority number	Risk reduction effort/ process improvement

When identifying risk-reduction efforts, select "hard-wired" actions rather than lower-impact actions. Hard-wired actions are forcing functions, such as installing engineering controls (e.g., lock-out functions on endoscopy decontamination equipment or barcoding labels on blood products), automation, and computerization. Examples of lower-impact actions, in descending order of impact include

- standardization and protocols
- checklists and double-check systems
- rules and policies
- education or information

Using lessons from human factors analysis, the more we can make it impossible to commit an error, the safer patient care will be. (See Figure 1.5 regarding high, medium, low–impact risk-reduction actions provided by the U.S. Pharmacopeia Center for the Advancement of Patient Safety.)

| Figure 1.5 | **High, Medium, Low-Impact Risk-Reduction Actions** |

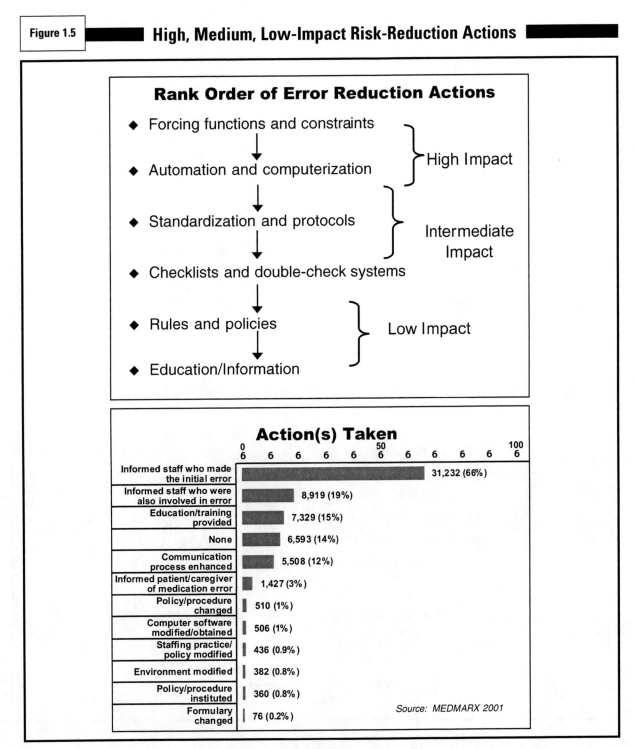

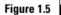 **High, Medium, Low-Impact Risk-Reduction Actions (cont.)**

Actions Taken Categorized Using Human Factors Analysis

Technical (Latent Error)	
Communication process enhanced	12
Computer software modified/obtained	1
Environment modified	0.8
Organizational (Latent Error)	
Environment modified	0.8
Formulary changed	0.2
Education/Training provided	15
Policy/procedure instituted	0.8
Policy/procedure changed	1
Staffing practice/policy modified	0.9
Human (Active Error)	
Communication process enhanced	12
Education/Training provided	15
Informed staff who made the initial error	66
Informed staff involved in the error	19
Patient	
Informed patient/caregiver of medication error	3
Other	
No action taken	14

Most prevalent

Strong Impact Actions (examples)

◆ Use engineering control or forcing function (e.g., IV tubing luer lock)

◆ Change architectural/physical plant (e.g., space for drug preparation, storage; lighting)

◆ Automate & computerize (e.g., drug dispensing; access to patient info, barcoding)

◆ Standardize equipment, processes, or protocols

◆ Simplify processes and remove unnecessary steps

◆ Involve leadership, support patient safety efforts

Figure 1.5 ▮▮▮ **High, Medium, Low-Impact Risk-Reduction Actions (cont.)** ▮▮▮

Intermediate Impact Actions (examples)

- ◆ Add software enhancements/modifications
- ◆ Create checklists
- ◆ Read back verbal orders
- ◆ Eliminate/reduce distractions (e.g., IV room)
- ◆ Cut redundancy
- ◆ Eliminate look-alike and sound-alike drugs
- ◆ Enhance documentation/communication

Weak Impact Actions (examples)

- ◆ Create new policy/procedure/memorandum
- ◆ Perform double checks
- ◆ Institute warnings and labels
- ◆ Provide training/education
- ◆ Assign additional study/analysis

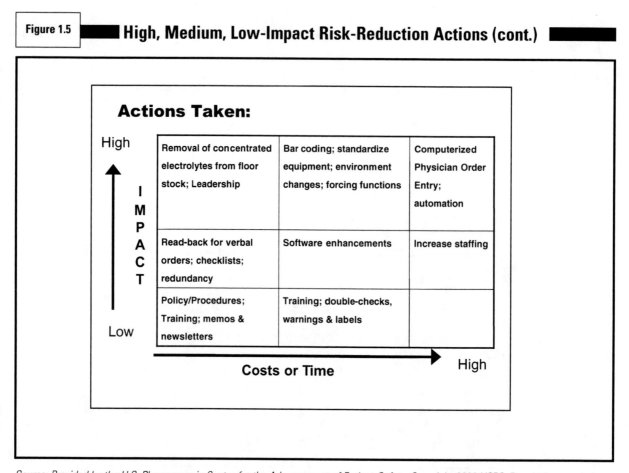

Source: Provided by the U.S. Pharmacopeia Center for the Advancement of Patient Safety, Copyright 2003 USPC. Permission granted.

From an organizational standpoint, the FMEA is beginning to move from the realm of risk management into the world of performance improvement. Treat the risk-reduction efforts as the organization treats its performance improvement efforts. Based upon the organization's method and approach toward performance improvement (e.g., Plan-Do-Check-Act or PDCA), the FMEA may begin to look different at this point. So that everyone in the organization can recognize it, fit the risk-reduction efforts into the organization's performance improvement methodology and use the tool in Figure 1.6 to track the effectiveness of the actions the team took to reduce risk.

Figure 1.6	■ Priorities for Risk-Reduction–Performance Improvement Process ■

Potential failure mode	Potential effect of failure mode	Risk priority number	Risk reduction strategies	Person(s) responsible for implementation	Planned date of implementation	Measurement strategy	Current status
Identify potential failures for each step in the process	Identify potential outcome of failure to patient						

8. **Test and carry out** the redesigned process before full-scale implementation. An essential element of performance improvement is to pilot test any improvement on a limited scale or targeted area of the organization prior to rolling it out organization-wide.

9. **Measure** the effectiveness of the redesigned process.

10. **Maintain** the effectiveness of the redesigned process.

The final two steps in the process are critical to the success of any performance improvement process. It is essential that organizations have a management process in place that ensures approved improvements are measured for effectiveness and maintained over time. If not, the organization will keep doing things the same way and continue to put patients at risk for future errors.

In addition to the evaluation of the steps in a process and how these steps inter-relate to create safe (or not-so-safe) practices, when conducting an FMEA, it is frequently valuable to look at the work environment within which that process occurs. The related article, "Examining how workspace affects patient safey," at the end of this chapter provides insight into how you would go about doing so.

CHAPTER 1

RELATED ARTICLES

EXAMINING HOW WORKSPACE AFFECTS PATIENT SAFETY

Expect accreditors and regulators to place more emphasis on how the physical design of your hospital's workspaces affects patient safety. A new report by the Institute of Medicine (IOM) strongly recommends that hospitals redesign their work processes and physical workspaces to make them more efficient, less vulnerable to errors, and more supportive to staff so they can detect and fix errors when they occur.

Background

A November 20, 2003, report marks the third time that the IOM has emphasized the inherent dangers of workspace design.

The IOM's 2000 exposé on medical errors, To Err is Human, recommended that hospitals and other health care organizations incorporate certain safety principles into work design.

A second report released in 2001, Crossing the Quality Chasm, said that "health care has safety and quality problems because it relies on outmoded systems of work. Poor designs set up the workforce to fail, regardless of how hard they try."

The latest report, Keeping Patients Safe: Transforming the Work Environment of Nurses, reiterates this, calling on facilities to retool their health care processes and create more thoughtful workspace design.

"Inefficient care processes and workspace design, while not intrinsically dangerous to patients, decrease patient safety to the extent that they reduce the time nurses have for monitoring patients and providing therapeutic care," wrote the IOM, a private nonprofit institution that provides health policy advice under a congressional charter granted to the National Academy of Sciences.

Tips and recommendations
The following pages highlight the IOM's recommendations.

EXAMINING HOW WORKSPACE AFFECTS PATIENT SAFETY (CONT.)

Examine workspace design

Think about your hospital's different units and the rooms and office areas that staff use every day to perform their work. How does this physical workspace help or hinder each staff member's ability to provide effective and safe patient care?

Five specific elements of the work system interact with each other and influence patient safety. Whenever one of them changes, all of the other elements are affected. The five elements include

1. the physical and professional characteristics of each staff member, such as the sensory, musculoskeletal, and cognitive skills required to perform certain tasks

2. the actual tasks performed and the characteristics that may contribute to unsafe patient care

3. the tools and technologies that staff use

4. the physical environment, such as the lighting, noise level, and distractions that can affect a health care provider's concentration and hinder patient safety

5. other processes and conditions within the organization, such hand-offs and how different units and departments communicate

Analyze work design

Analyze how your workspaces and work design affect patient safety using one of the following techniques:

1. **Work sampling:** A growing number of hospitals use this method to learn how nursing staff spend their time, and to identify problems within each unit's workspace design. It involves observing staff several times at random or fixed intervals and documenting all tasks that they perform during each observation.

EXAMINING HOW WORKSPACE AFFECTS PATIENT SAFETY (CONT.)

Note: The IOM doesn't favor this method. It says work sampling observations are limited because they don't accurately reflect all of the work that a nurse does on a given unit or in a given space. "The method assumes that the tasks involved are observable, unambiguous, mutually exclusive, and exhaustive—not always the case with much of nursing work," the IOM states.

2. **Root-cause analyses (RCAs):** Conduct these after an error or adverse event. They can help you prevent them from happening again. RCAs answer several questions, including the following:

   - What happened?
   - Why did it happen?
   - What were the factors that caused it to happen?
   - Why did those factors occur?
   - What systems and processes underlie those factors?

3. **FMEA:** Unlike RCAs, hospitals can use FMEAs before errors occur to identify vulnerable areas and develop strategies and processes for avoiding them.

Get direct input from frontline staff

Analyze and design work processes with active involvement from the nursing staff.

"Employee participation is a key ingredient in successful organizational change, improving the outcome of work redesign, and facilitating its successful implementation," the IOM states.

The IOM is careful to distinguish that active participation is preferable because it allows staff to directly identify problems and solutions.

Passive participation, on the other hand, merely involves telling staff about upcoming changes to their workspace without seeking their input or suggestions.

EXAMINING HOW WORKSPACE AFFECTS PATIENT SAFETY (CONT.)

Each nursing unit, for example, is organized differently and in accordance with things such as patient population, management approaches, work allocation, resources, and experience level of its nurses.

A unit with highly experienced nurses, therefore, may need a different structure than one with novice nurses. As the nurses' work changes, so should the structure of the unit and how it is organized and managed.

Simplify and standardize common work procedures and equipment

The use of clinical pathways, for example, is one way to standardize patient care to reduce variation and a provider's reliance on memory.

"Simplifying and standardizing routine procedures, such as IV insertion, catheter insertion, dressing changes, tracheotomy care, and other nursing treatments and procedures, minimizes opportunities for slips and lapses," says the IOM.

A standardized room design, therefore, might have all electrical outlets located in a certain area or standardize the way that medical supplies are stocked throughout the hospital.

"Such standardization of patient care environments and equipment decreases the cognitive load on nurses, making slips and lapses less likely to occur during routine tasks by minimizing decision time and manipulation time," states the IOM.

Decrease interruptions, distractions, and interferences

Understanding the following definitions will help you decrease these three problems:

- An **interruption** is defined as the "cessation of a task" before it has been completed due to an external factor.

- A **distraction** is an "external stimulus" that causes a human response, but not the cessation of the task.

- **Interference** includes competition for the cognitive resources required to perform simultaneous tasks. Errors attributed to interference are more likely to occur with new or difficult tasks.

All three elements are common in health care and pose significant danger to patient safety. In fact, nurses cite distractions and interruptions as chief contributors to medication errors, while health professionals cite all three as the primary causes of medical errors in general.

Consider this: Nearly 80% of licensed nurses in Illinois and North Carolina agree that "tasks are often interrupted without being completed," according to a survey conducted by the National Institute for Occupational Safety and Health (NIOSH) of the U.S. Centers for Disease Control and Prevention.

TIP: Hospitals should determine where nurses and other health care providers are most distracted and redesign the workspace or work processes to reduce those distractions. This is particularly important on the intensive care unit, where noise from clinical alarms and medical equipment can become so common that nurses filter it out.

This is one reason why the National Patient Safety Goals of the JCAHO requires hospitals to improve the effectiveness of clinical alarm systems, by ensuring that nurses can hear them amid competing noise on the unit.

Create redundancy and back-up systems

Build repetition directly into your hospital's work processes so that staff are trained to react automatically and will easily notice when something is out of place or has been completed incorrectly.

To do this, use "forcing functions" that prevent staff from making an erroneous action.

EXAMINING HOW WORKSPACE AFFECTS PATIENT SAFETY (CONT.)

A computerized physician order entry system, for example, is a forcing function that requires physicians to enter certain information onto their order before the computer will accept and process it.

"When [your organization] spends the money to create redundancy, there is no question that it takes the possibility of errors very seriously," the IOM states.

Don't rely on one staff member's vigilance

Since your workers cannot maintain high-intensity vigilance over prolonged periods, don't rely on them to do so to monitor safety threats, the IOM said.

Alarms on automatic IV pumps and other patient monitoring devices, for example, allow patients and their family members to monitor their equipment.

"When patients and their families are knowledgeable about certain treatment protocols and prescribed medications, they can take a more active role in monitoring care, as well as providing self-care," the IOM concluded.

Improve information access

Information technology can reduce work errors and inefficiencies and increase patient safety.

In its report, the IOM described the automated patient record system employed by Intermountain Health Care (IHC) in Salt Lake City. IHC allows staff to access patient histories, physical exams, vital signs, allergy information, lab test results, and other clinical data online. The system's other benefits include the following:

- **Organized, legible data:** Nurses can see all of the prescribed drugs for a patient in one location. The doses are written clearly, names are spelled correctly, and data are grouped to ensure that important information is easy to locate. In addition, other members of the patient's health care team can view the nurse's concerns and respond to them.

EXAMINING HOW WORKSPACE AFFECTS PATIENT SAFETY (CONT.)

- **Support for ongoing knowledge acquisition:** The hospital can link the patient's clinical data to reference literature to answer questions about policies, procedures, prognoses, diagnoses, educational materials, appropriate drug doses, and drug contraindications.

- **The system can alert staff to changes and can flag nurses with reminders:** For patients who take the medication Coumadin, IHC's computer system shows the results of the most recent clotting factor test or the absence of such critical results so that staff can see which patients are out of acceptable blood value ranges and need dosage adjustments or another test.

For patients with diabetes, the system flags those patients who are due for glycosalated hemoglobin tests and retinal exams, for example. The system sends out similar alerts and reminders regarding pap smears, mammograms, and immunizations.

Use an FMEA to identify workspace problems

Performing an FMEA is one of your most powerful and proactive patient safety tools, particularly because FMEAs allow you to identify weaknesses and unsafe practices before they cause harm to patients.

FMEAs were developed in the 1960s to improve safety in the aerospace industry. They were widely applied to the health care industry in 2001 when the JCAHO began requiring accredited organizations to perform at least one proactive risk assessment each year.

The term "failure mode" typically refers to a vulnerability within a hospital's processes that can result in harm to a patient. The goal of an FMEA is to prevent errors from occurring by doing the following:

- Identifying all of the ways a process or device can fail
- Estimating the probability and consequence of each failure
- Taking action to prevent the potential failures from occurring

---

EXAMINING HOW WORKSPACE AFFECTS PATIENT SAFETY (CONT.)

You do not need to conduct FMEAs on all processes, however. Sometimes, you may focus on the physical workspace itself.

Don't use short-term FMEA fixes

There are two ways to address a problem identified through your FMEA: The right way and the wrong way.

The wrong way gives you weak-impact solutions that lose their effectiveness over time as staff slip back into their old habits.

Consider new training and education, double-checks, or new policies and procedures. True, each of these measures is helpful, but alone, not one is enough to permanently address the kinds of systemic problems that are usually identified through a FMEA, says John Santell, MS, RPh, director of educational program initiatives at U.S. Pharmacopeia's Center for the Advancement of Patient Safety.

Instead, your hospital should employ a combination of strong-, intermediate-, and weak-impact actions to yield long-term results, says Santell, who spoke with other experts during a recent HCPro-sponsored audioconference, "Medication Management: How to use FMEA to identify high-risk areas in your system."

Strong-impact actions
Strong-impact actions have a lasting effect because they address problems on a broad level and are often so sweeping that they become forced changes that staff don't even have to think about. Examples include

- using automated drug dispensing
- employing engineering controls, such as an IV tubing lock or bar coding
- making architectural changes to the workspace, such by redesigning the spaces that staff use to prepare or store drugs
- removing unnecessary steps in the medication administration processes
- getting leadership to take action and visibly support all patient safety efforts

EXAMINING HOW WORKSPACE AFFECTS PATIENT SAFETY (CONT.)

Intermediate-impact actions

Intermediate-impact actions are often more tempting than high-impact solutions because they require fewer resources and can be implemented more quickly. But like weak impact actions, they aren't quite enough to produce lasting, system-wide changes. Examples include

- eliminating look-alike or sound-alike drug names
- developing checklists
- reducing noise and distractions
- enhancing documentation or communication procedures

If your hospital's FMEA uncovers potential problems in the medication ordering process and it decides to require physicians to use generic names on medication orders, the pharmacy team might

- develop a new policy that allows pharmacists to refuse to fill orders that don't include the drug's indication and brand and generic names
- meet with medical staff leaders to get their full backing
- send out memos to alert physicians of the change
- use warning labels on certain look-alike or sound-alike drugs
- research options for using a computerized physician order entry system
- print out a formulary/drug list that includes each drug's brand name, generic name, pharmacologic category, and dose/strength to help physicians and nurses learn drug names, and place the list in each medication cart and medication room

Crucial: Make sure the senior leadership and medical staff support the policy. Physicians might not want to change their practices immediately, but hospital leadership must support the pharmacy in saying it will not accept orders unless the drug's generic name is on them.

In addition, the pharmacy team might hold regular staff meetings to discuss its risk-reduction efforts.

Editor's note: Visit www.iom.edu/reports.asp *to obtain a copy of the new IOM report. To obtain a cassette tape of the November 19, 2003, audioconference, "Medication Management: How to use FMEA to identify high-risk areas in your system," call customer service at 800/ 650-6787.*

Source: *Examining how workspace affects patient safety,* Briefings on Patient Safety, *special report, January 2004, HCPro, Inc.*

USE FMEAS FOR MORE THAN JUST REGULATORY COMPLIANCE, EXPERTS ADVISE

For some organizations, conducting an FMEA is something they do just to comply with the JCAHO standards. But when done correctly, the process can help you improve patient care and safety.

FMEAs can help your facility correct potential problems, said Craig Clapper, chief operating officer of Performance Improvement International of San Clemente, CA, during an audioconference hosted by HCPro, Inc.

To benefit from the tool, conduct FMEAs on a regular basis. That means you need to convince leaders in your center that the analysis is a valuable part of your quality program, said Clapper. Demonstrate that your center will save money if procedures are safer and more efficient. Some centers see a 50% reduction in production costs as a result of adopting corrective actions after conducting an FMEA, Clapper said.

Using an FMEA correctly

An FMEA identifies potential high-risk behaviors and situations before a sentinel event occurs. A root-cause analysis, on the other hand, analyzes a sentinel event and helps organizations prevent the same thing from happening again, said Robert Marder, MD, practice director of quality and patient safety at The Greeley Company, a division of HCPro, Inc. Marder also spoke during the audioconference.

The first step in conducting an FMEA is identifying a high-risk process and breaking it down into its various steps. For example, giving a patient his or her medication involves identifying the patient and correctly using the medication administration record, said Clapper. Analyzing each step will help you better spot potential problems.

If you only conduct an FMEA once or twice per year to comply with JCAHO standards, the process will seem difficult and frustrating, says Marder. The more frequently you do the analysis, the easier the process will become and you will be able to correct more potential problem areas. But focus first on learning to use the tool correctly, advised Marder.

"You don't need another bad analysis. What you need is a good one that helps you improve," he said.

Use FMEAs for more than just regulatory compliance, experts advise (cont.)

Look at failures in each step

One example of a process you can break down into smaller steps is identifying patients, says Marder.

Properly identifying the patient includes comparing the name and date of birth on the medical record chart with the same information on the patient's wrist-band, confirming the information with the patient, and checking to make sure that the physician and patient agree why the patient needs treatment.

Each step in a process can potentially result in failure, said Clapper. When trying to come up with different ways in which the steps can fail, consult clinical members of your staff. They will have first-hand experience with problem areas.

You can also use a list of different positions, actions, and consequences to help you identify more failure modes.

"Don't come up with just one failure mode for a given activity," says Marder said. "You should always have at least two failure modes, either something didn't occur or something happened that was incorrect. If you think of more ways to fail, you are more likely to find opportunities for improvement."

For example, a clerk could incorrectly fill out the patient's name on the medication record, or perhaps the physician compared the medical record with the patient's wristband, but didn't ask the patient whether the information was correct.

"If you think a failure mode couldn't happen, another facility has probably already experienced it," said Clapper.

Correcting the problems

When you outline ways to correct different problems, take into account that some errors occur when staff are in a rush, and some happen because staff either don't know your policies or choose to ignore them. Don't take a "one-size-fits-all approach" to correcting errors, advises Marder.

Use FMEAs for more than just regulatory compliance, experts advise (cont.)

Once you conduct an FMEA and establish and implement corrective actions, recalculate the different RPNs to see whether the number decreased.If you find the error is less likely to happen or the outcome is less severe, then you know the FMEA has had a positive impact on your organization, said Clapper.

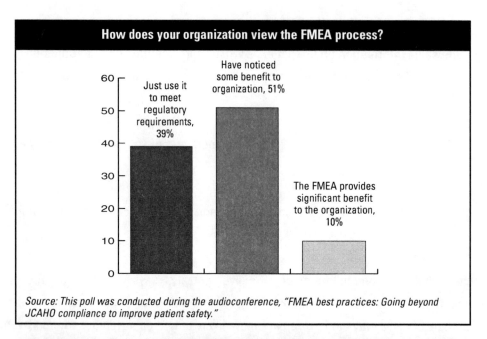

How does your organization view the FMEA process?

Source: This poll was conducted during the audioconference, "FMEA best practices: Going beyond JCAHO compliance to improve patient safety."

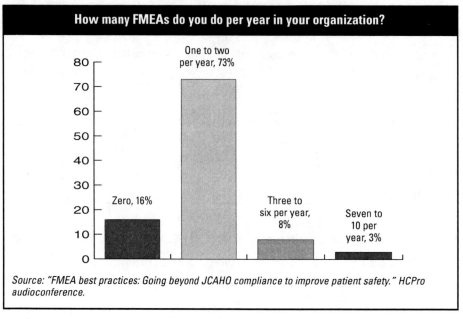

How many FMEAs do you do per year in your organization?

Source: "FMEA best practices: Going beyond JCAHO compliance to improve patient safety." HCPro audioconference.

Source: Briefings on Ambulatory Accreditation, *August 2003, HCPro, Inc.*

Chapter 2

CASE STUDY:
BLOOD TRANSFUSION FMEA

CHAPTER 2

Case Study: Blood Transfusion FMEA

Blood transfusion errors are among the top 10 sentinel events that have occurred at accredited organizations since the Joint Commission on Accreditation of Healthcare Organizations (JCAHO) started reviewing sentinel events in 1995.

For the sake of this case study, we will define a transfusion error as a complication of blood transfusion where there is an immune response against the transfused blood cells or other components of the transfusion. Generally speaking, health care organizations have built several steps into the blood transfusion process to significantly reduce the risk of blood transfusion error, including the following:

- Confirming multiple patient identifiers during the various stages of the transfusion process

- Typing donated blood into ABO and Rh groups prior to a transfusion

- Cross-matching to further confirm that the blood is compatible (during the cross-matching process, a small amount of donor blood is mixed with a small amount of recipient blood and the mixture is examined under a microscope for signs of antibody reaction)

Despite these universally accepted industry-wide efforts, transfusion reactions continue to occur. The immediate cause of most blood transfusion errors (what has been referred to as "the sharp end" of the process) is a failure at the bedside to detect that an incorrect unit of blood has been issued. A significant contributing factor to such errors (much earlier in the process) is misidentification of lab specimens.

Blood transfusions represent one of the more complex processes in health care institutions today due to the large number of hand-offs between multiple health care providers representing different disciplines and departments. This complexity, coupled with the significant communication that is involved in the process, makes blood transfusion an excellent target for Failure Modes and Effects Analysis (FMEA).

Using the process outlined in Chapter 1, we now will follow the FMEA of the blood transfusion process, step by step. The ultimate goal of this FMEA is to reduce the risk of a devastating blood transfusion error occurring within an organization.

Step 1: Organize the team

Based upon the ultimate objective of reducing the risk of blood transfusion errors and using the strategy explained in Chapter 1, the organization's leaders selected the following staff to participate in this FMEA:

Core FMEA team members:

- Administrative director, laboratory
- Chief of pathology
- Blood bank supervisor
- Chief nursing officer
- Clinical manager, emergency department
- Nursing supervisor
- Risk manager, facilitator

Ad-hoc team members:

- Registered nurse, emergency department
- Registered nurse, intensive care unit
- Registered nurse, operating room
- Safety officer
- Director, information systems
- Director, plant operations
- Licensed practical nurse, medical/surgical

Step 2: Flowchart the process

Using software, the team flowcharted the entire blood administration process, which appears in Figure 2.1 beginning on the following page.

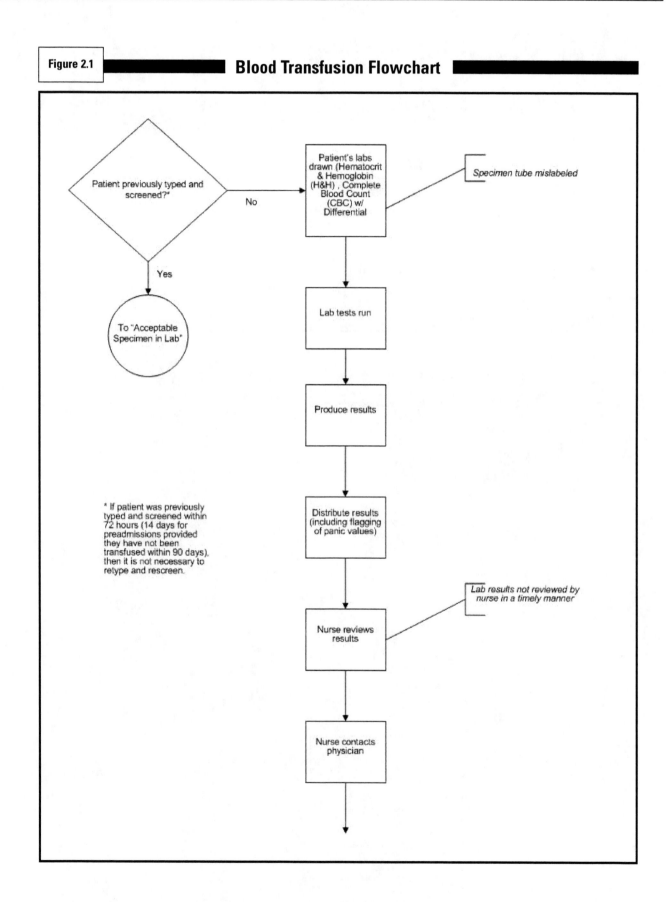

Figure 2.1   **Blood Transfusion Flowchart**

Patient previously typed and screened?*

No

Yes

To "Acceptable Specimen in Lab"

Patient's labs drawn (Hematocrit & Hemoglobin (H&H) , Complete Blood Count (CBC) w/ Differential

Specimen tube mislabeled

Lab tests run

Produce results

* If patient was previously typed and screened within 72 hours (14 days for preadmissions provided they have not been transfused within 90 days), then it is not necessary to retype and rescreen.

Distribute results (including flagging of panic values)

Lab results not reviewed by nurse in a timely manner

Nurse reviews results

Nurse contacts physician

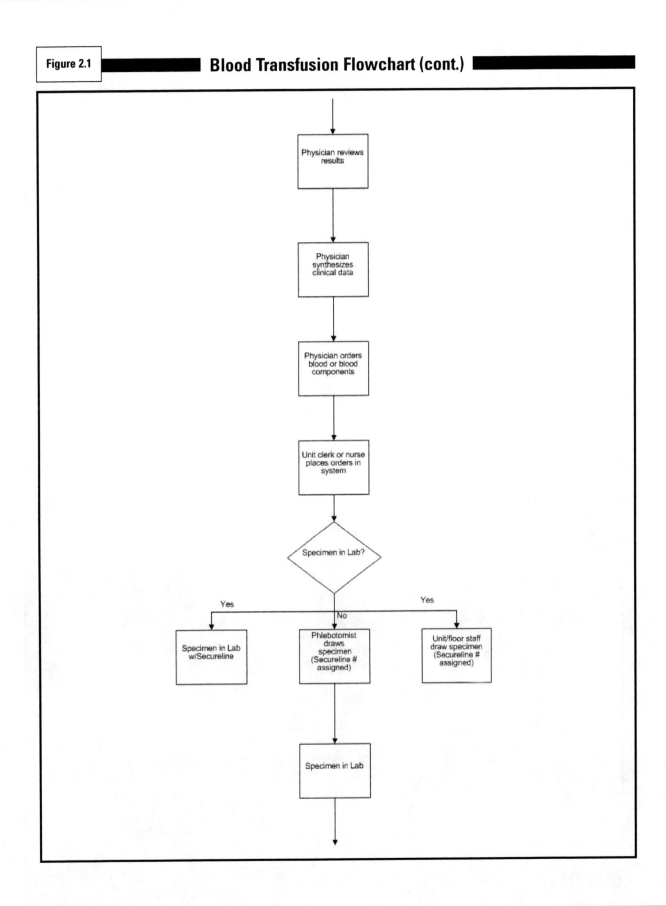

Figure 2.1 — Blood Transfusion Flowchart (cont.)

Figure 2.1 ████████ **Blood Transfusion Flowchart (cont.)** ████████

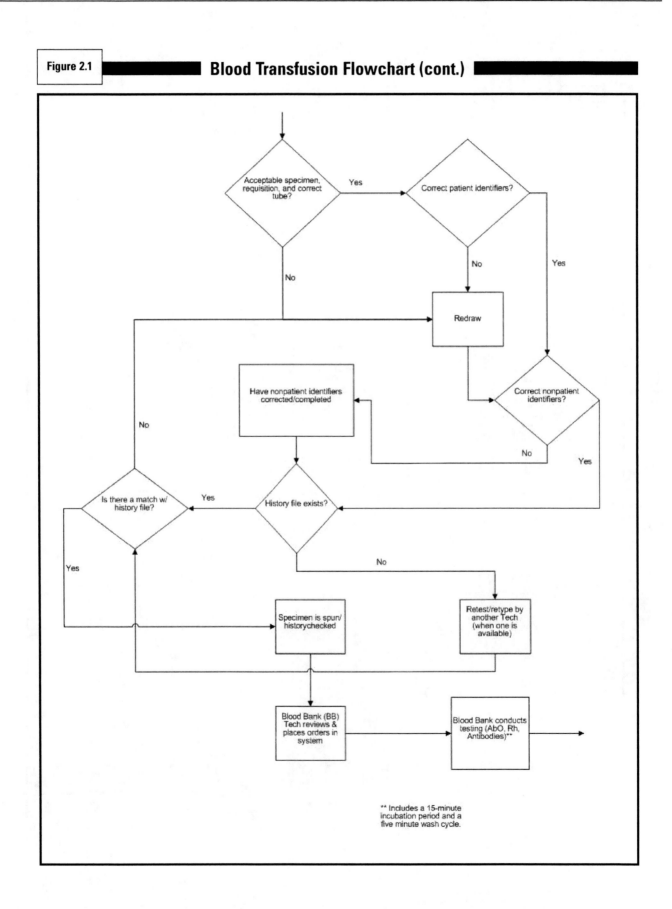

** Includes a 15-minute
incubation period and a
five minute wash cycle.

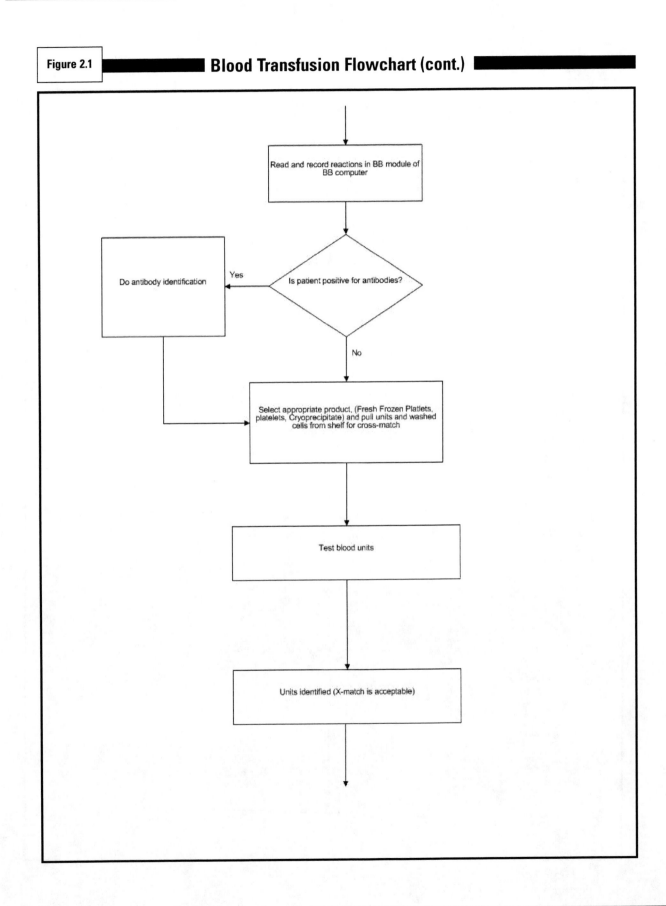

Figure 2.1   **Blood Transfusion Flowchart (cont.)**

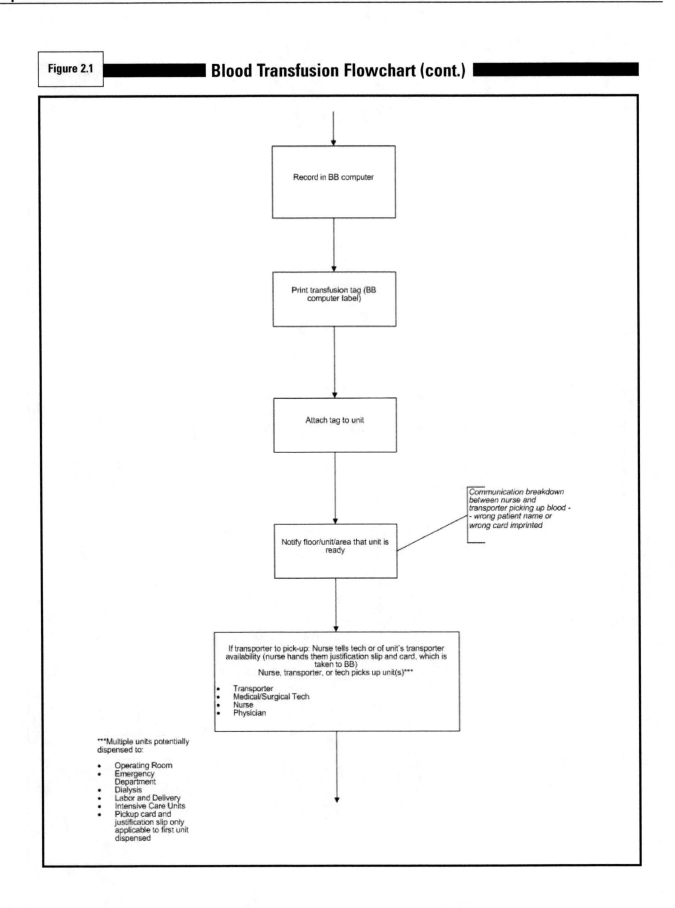

Figure 2.1 **Blood Transfusion Flowchart (cont.)**

Record in BB computer

Print transfusion tag (BB computer label)

Attach tag to unit

Notify floor/unit/area that unit is ready

Communication breakdown between nurse and transporter picking up blood -- wrong patient name or wrong card imprinted

If transporter to pick-up: Nurse tells tech or of unit's transporter availability (nurse hands them justification slip and card, which is taken to BB)
Nurse, transporter, or tech picks up unit(s)***

- Transporter
- Medical/Surgical Tech
- Nurse
- Physician

***Multiple units potentially dispensed to:

- Operating Room
- Emergency Department
- Dialysis
- Labor and Delivery
- Intensive Care Units
- Pickup card and justification slip only applicable to first unit dispensed

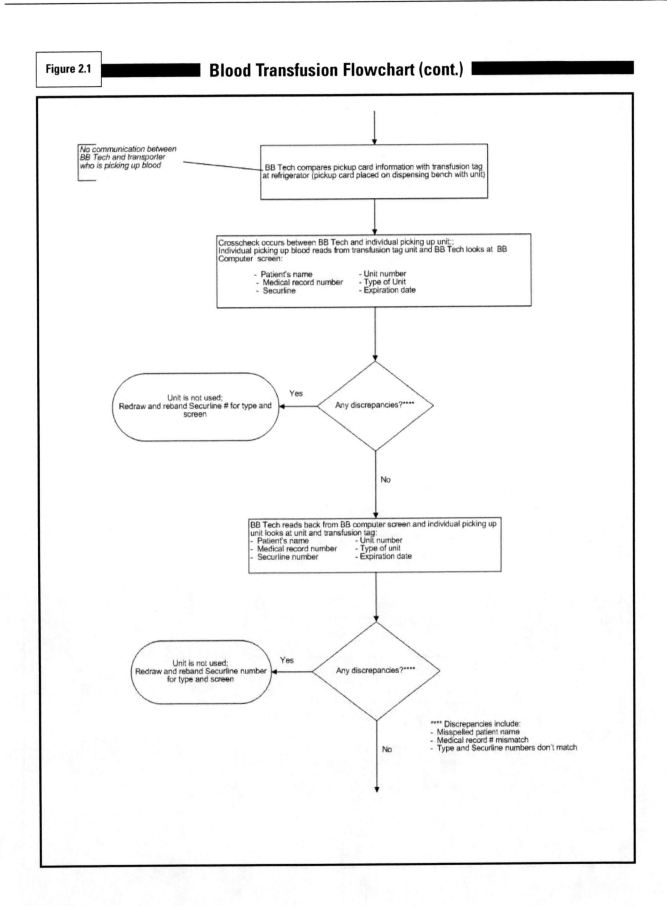

Figure 2.1 **Blood Transfusion Flowchart (cont.)**

No communication between BB Tech and transporter who is picking up blood

BB Tech compares pickup card information with transfusion tag at refrigerator (pickup card placed on dispensing bench with unit)

Crosscheck occurs between BB Tech and individual picking up unit:;
Individual picking up blood reads from transfusion tag unit and BB Tech looks at BB Computer screen:

- Patient's name
- Medical record number
- Securline
- Unit number
- Type of Unit
- Expiration date

Any discrepancies?****

Yes → Unit is not used; Redraw and reband Securline # for type and screen

No ↓

BB Tech reads back from BB computer screen and individual picking up unit looks at unit and transfusion tag:
- Patient's name
- Medical record number
- Securline number
- Unit number
- Type of unit
- Expiration date

Any discrepancies?****

Yes → Unit is not used; Redraw and reband Securline number for type and screen

No ↓

**** Discrepancies include:
- Misspelled patient name
- Medical record # mismatch
- Type and Securline numbers don't match

Figure 2.1 ██████████ **Blood Transfusion Flowchart (cont.)** ██████████

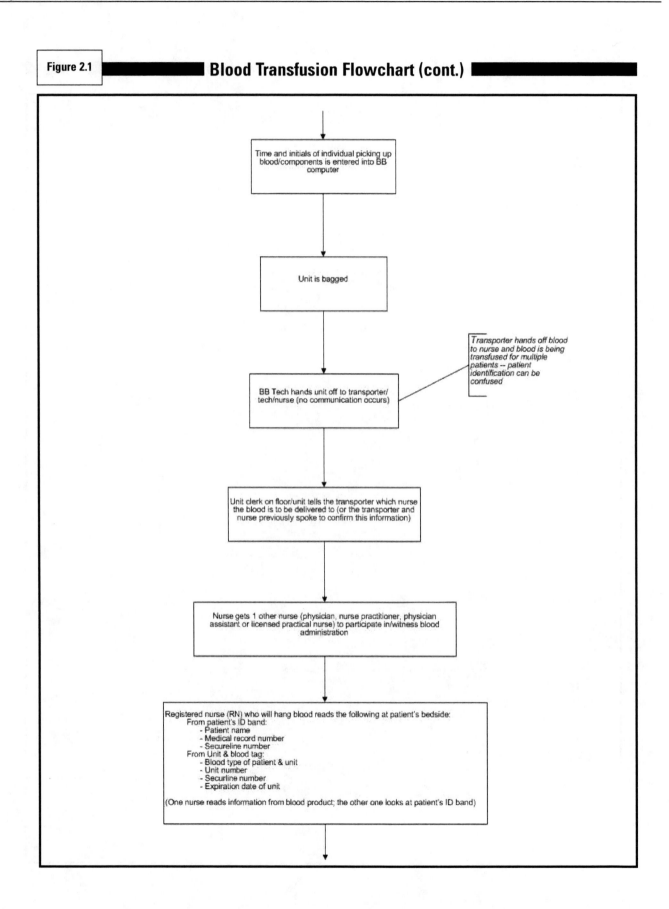

Time and initials of individual picking up blood/components is entered into BB computer

Unit is bagged

BB Tech hands unit off to transporter/ tech/nurse (no communication occurs)

Transporter hands off blood to nurse and blood is being transfused for multiple patients -- patient identification can be confused

Unit clerk on floor/unit tells the transporter which nurse the blood is to be delivered to (or the transporter and nurse previously spoke to confirm this information)

Nurse gets 1 other nurse (physician, nurse practitioner, physician assistant or licensed practical nurse) to participate in/witness blood administration

Registered nurse (RN) who will hang blood reads the following at patient's bedside:
  From patient's ID band:
        - Patient name
        - Medical record number
        - Secureline number
  From Unit & blood tag:
        - Blood type of patient & unit
        - Unit number
        - Securline number
        - Expiration date of unit

(One nurse reads information from blood product; the other one looks at patient's ID band)

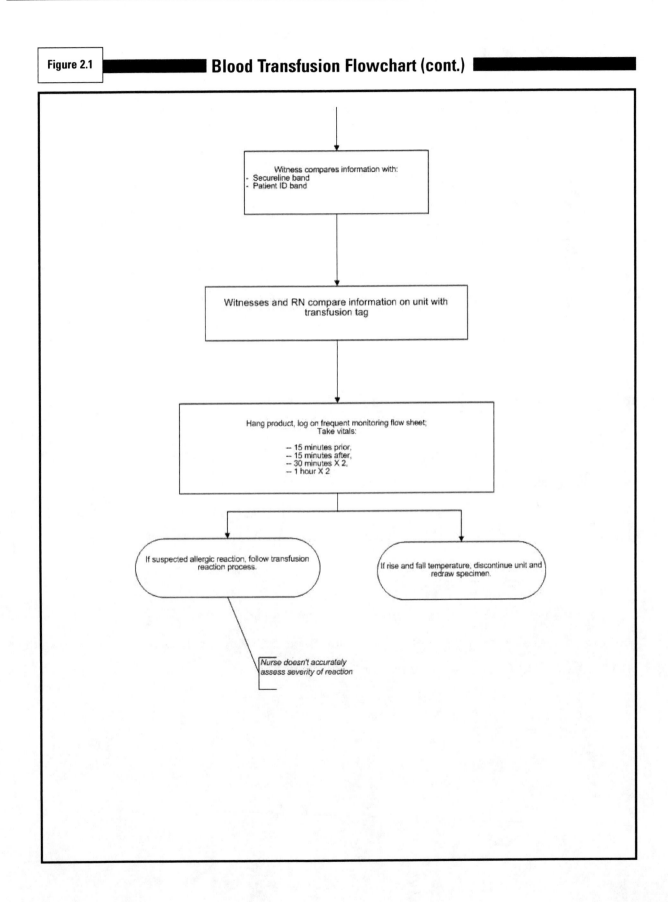

Figure 2.1 Blood Transfusion Flowchart (cont.)

Step 3: Identify potential failure modes

The facilitator then led the FMEA team through a review of the finalized flowchart to identify individual steps in the process that might be vulnerable to break down. These potential failure modes were then added to the flowchart in Figure 2.1 (for readability, not all of the failure modes that were identified by the FMEA team are affixed to the flowchart).

The potential failure modes during the process include mislabeled specimen tubes, delayed reviews of lab results, or communication breakdowns between the nurse and transporter picking up blood. The potential failure modes were then entered into the matrix described in Chapter 1, and the group reached agreement on the frequency, severity, and detectability of the individual failure modes. From there, the team computed the risk priority number.

Step 4: Identify the potential effect of each failure mode

For each of the potential failure modes, the team identified the ultimate impact on the patient. For example, the team determined it was likely that a patient would be harmed if there is a communication breakdown between the nurse and the transporter picking up the blood. It rated the potential for harm as a 10 (on a scale of 1–10) if, as a result of the communication breakdown, the transporter picks up the wrong patient's blood.

However, the team determined that there was a very minor chance (a score of 1) that a patient would be harmed if, as a result of the physician order for blood not being timely, that there would be a delay in the transfusion. See Figure 2.2 for the completed FMEA matrix.

Figure 2.2 **Completed FMEA Matrix**

COMMUNITY HOSPITAL
FAILURE MODE AND EFFECTS ANALYSIS
PRIVILEGED AND CONFIDENTIAL

PROCESS TO BE ASSESSED: **Blood Transfusion**

Potential failure mode	Potential effect of failure mode	Frequency (Likeliness scale) 1–10	Severity (Potential for harm) 1–10	Detectability (Potential discovery) 1–10	Risk priority number
Identify potential failures for each step in the process	Identify potential outcome of failure to patient	On a scale of 1 – 10 (10 = highly likely), identify the likelihood of this failure actually occurring Example: 1 = Remote probability 5 = Moderate probability 10 = Very high probability	On a scale of 1 – 10 (10 = worst potential failure outcome), identify the potential severity of the consequences of this failure Example: 1 = Very minor outcome 5 = Moderate outcome 10 = Very severe outcome	On a scale of 1 – 10 (1 = failure easily discovered under normal circumstances) highly likely), identify the potential difficulty of discovery of failure Example: 1 = Certain detection 5 = Possible detection 10 = Cannot detect	RPN = Frequency X Severity X Detectability
At time of blood pick-up in Blood Bank – no communication between Blood Bank Tech & transporter who is picking up blood	Wrong patient's blood is handed off from Blood Bank Tech to transporter	9	10	10	900
Communication breakdown between nurse & transporter picking up blood —wrong patient name	Wrong patient's blood is requested from Blood Bank	9	10	10	900
Communication breakdown between nurse & transporter picking up blood —wrong card imprinted	Wrong patient's blood is requested from Blood Bank	9	10	10	900
Lab results not reviewed by nurse in a timely manner	Patient's need for blood transfusion is delayed	5	8	10	400
Transporter hands off blood to nurse & blood is being transfused for multiple patients - patient identification can be confused	Patient receives wrong blood	4	10	10	400

Figure 2.2	Completed FMEA Matrix (cont.)

Failure Mode	Effect				RPN
Nurse doesn't accurately assess severity of reaction	Patient's reaction goes unnoticed	5	10	8	400
Specimen tube mislabeled	Wrong patient's blood is typed and cross-matched	3	10	10	300
Delay in blood specimen transport to Lab	Blood specimen can't be processed – delay in transfusion	5	5	7	175
Blood Bank Tech distracted during testing blood unit – inaccurate results	Mix-up in patient's type and cross-match	4	7	5	140
Illegible transfusion tag	Wrong blood type transfused	3	7	6	126
Specimen not viable	Delay in blood transfusion	3	8	5	120
Blood order entered on wrong patient	Wrong blood type cross-matched	3	8	5	120
Phlebotomist draws wrong patient's specimen	Patient receives wrong blood type	2	10	5	100
Transfusion reaction – physician doesn't call back	Delay in treating transfusion	9	10	1	90
Inaccurate transfusion tag on blood	Patient receives wrong blood type	1	9	9	81
Blood Bank Tech doesn't check specimen tube upon arrival in Blood Bank	Delay in treating transfusion	4	5	4	80
Blood Bank Tech doesn't check requisition upon arrival in Blood Bank	Delay in treating transfusion	4	5	4	80
Lab results not communicated to physician	Patient's need for blood transfusion is delayed	3	5	5	75
Blood Bank Tech enters wrong blood type into computer system	Patient receives wrong blood type	1	8	8	64

Figure 2.2		Completed FMEA Matrix (cont.)			
Blood Bank Tech places blood pick-up card on bench/doesn't use it to match up with product at refrigerator	Patient receives wrong blood type	3	5	3	45
Blood Bank Tech picks out wrong unit from refrigerator	Patient receives wrong blood type	3	5	3	45
Transcription error on the original blood order	Patient receives wrong blood type	2	5	4	40
Transfusion tag is detached from unit during administration	Unable to confirm that patient received correct blood	5	8	1	40
Duplicate orders for type and cross	Confusion in Blood Bank – multiple specimens mixed-up	6	6	1	36
Delay in notifying floor that blood is ready	Delay in transfusion	3	4	3	36
Lab instrument not calibrated	Inaccurate blood typing and cross-matches	1	7	5	35
Lab test results inaccurate	Inaccurate blood typing and cross-matches	1	5	5	25
Old Securline band not removed	Confusion leading to delay in transfusion	5	5	1	25
Physician doesn't answer calls re: lab results	Delay in transfusion	5	5	1	25
Delay in blood order entry	Delay in transfusion	1	5	5	25
Blood Bank Tech workload heavy during testing blood unit – inaccurate results	Wrong blood transfused	3	5	1	15
Delay in blood pickup from Blood Bank	Delay in transfusion	2	5	1	10
Physician order for blood not clear	Need to clarify order — delay in transfusion	2	3	1	6
Phlebotomist forgets to assign Securline number	Delay in transfusion	1	6	1	6

Figure 2.2 Completed FMEA Matrix (cont.)

Physician order for blood not timed	Unable to confirm timeliness of transfusion— delay in transfusion	5	1	1	5
Delay in nurse hanging unit	Delay in transfusion	1	5	1	5
Wrong patient on consent	Delay in transfusion	2	2	1	4
Delayed response by physician re: labs	Delay in transfusion	2	2	1	4
No consent	Delay in transfusion	2	1	1	2
Computer system is down – delayed lab results	Delay in transfusion	1	2	1	2
Computer system is down – delayed blood order	Delay in transfusion	1	2	1	2
Computer system is down – delayed blood typing	Delay in transfusion	1	2	1	2

Step 5: Redesign the processes/underlying systems

The next step was to brainstorm potential improvements to the existing processes to reduce the risk of the processes breaking down and negatively affecting the patient. For example, the team came up with several ideas to reduce the risk of a communication breakdown between the nurse and the transporter. The organization revised its process so that a direct hand-off of the blood card occurs at the nurses' station between the nurse who transfuses the blood/blood product and the nurse transporter who picks it up. However, the hand-off only occurs after the nurse transporter enters the patient's name, medical record number, and type of product being picked up into the transportation log. The blood/ blood product is then hand delivered to the nurse who hangs the product. See Figure 2.3 for the complete results of this brainstorming activity.

Figure 2.3	Blood Transfusion Risk-Reduction Efforts

Community Hospital

Failure Modes and Effects Analysis

Privileged and Confidential

Process to be assessed: Blood transfusion

Potential failure mode	Responsible party	Risk priority number (RPN)	Process improvement/risk-reduction effort
1. Blood pick-up—no communication between blood bank tech and transporter.	Blood bank supervisor	900	**Revised process** 1. Transporter presents pick-up card and states that he/she is there to pick up patient X's blood product (specify the product). 2. Blood bank tech inspects pick-up card and confirms that the following information is present on the card: <ul><li>Patient name</li><li>Medical record number</li><li>Vital signs</li><li>Securline number</li></ul> 3. Blood bank tech pulls up the patient information in computer and hands the card back to the transporter who then reads: <ul><li>Patient name</li><li>Medical record number</li><li>Securline number</li></ul>Blood bank tech compares each piece of information one at a time with the information on computer, using confirmatory communication, such as, "that is correct" or "that is wrong." 4. Blood bank tech takes the card and retrieves the appropriate blood or blood product. 5. Blood bank tech hands the blood or blood product to the transporter.

Figure 2.3 ██████ **Blood Transfusion Risk-Reduction Efforts (cont.)** ██████

			6. Transporter reads the following from the blood transfusion tag: • Patient name • Medical record number • Securline number • Patient blood type • Unit number • Unit blood type • Expiration date The blood bank tech compares the information with that on computer and, using active (not passive) confirmation, confirms each item's match one at a time. 7. The unit is signed out and released. **New rule (or formalize and reinforce existing rule)** 1. Only one unit of blood is processed at a time. **Next steps** 1. Revise blood release/distribution policy. 2. Educate all applicable staff regarding official new process. 3. Monitor for compliance.
Communication breakdown between nurse and transporter. Transporter picks up product labeled with the wrong patient name.	Transportation supervisor	900	**Revised process** 1. A direct hand-off of the blood card must occur at the nurses' station between the nurse who transfuses the blood or blood product and the transporter who picks up the blood or blood product. 2. This hand-off occurs only after the nurse transporter has entered the patient's name, medical record number, and type of product being picked up into the transportation log. 3. The blood or blood product is then hand-delivered to the nurse who hangs the product.

Figure 2.3 ████ Blood Transfusion Risk-Reduction Efforts (cont.) ████

			Next steps
			1. Revise the blood administration policy accordingly.
			2. Investigate the option of having the pick-up card printed by computer and being part of the transfusion tag (a multi-part form).
3. Communication breakdown between nurse and transporter picking up blood—wrong card imprinted.	Nurse clinical manager, Med/Surgical	900	After the card is imprinted (*but prior to issuing the card to the transporter*), the nurse goes to the patient bedside and compares the two official hospital patient identifiers (patient name and medical record number) on the card and the patient's identification band.
4. Lab results not reviewed by nurse in a timely manner.	Nursing clinical manager, intensive care unit (ICU)	400	1. For blood or blood products going to the operating room, labor and delivery, and emergency room on a stat basis, the blood bank calls the floor when blood is ready for pick-up.
			2. Change computer to provide unit-specific census information (only allow each unit to retrieve a list of the patients on their unit or default the initial listing to just the unit in question, rather than the entire house as with the former system).
			3. Re-educate unit secretarial staff on the use of the panic value form on the floor with a read-back from the unit secretary to the lab tech on the actual value.
5. Transporter/tech hands off blood to nurse and blood is transfused for multiple patients—patient identification can be confused.	Transportation supervisor	400	As in #2 above, the blood or blood product will be hand-delivered by the transporter to the nurse who will administer the blood or blood product.
7. Nurse doesn't accurately assess severity of reaction.	Nursing education director	400	Develop a checklist of the signs and symptoms of transfusion reaction used when administering blood. Checklist should include an algorithm that provides direction, such as action to be taken in response to a reaction.

Figure 2.3 ■■■■■ **Blood Transfusion Risk-Reduction Efforts (cont.)** ■■■■■

8. Specimen tube mislabeled.	Lab administrative director	300	**Revised process**
			
			Enter order into computer
			
			V
			
			Print and retrieve label
			
			V
			
			Draw specimen
			
			V
			
			Apply label (addressograph or computer-generated) at bedside
			
			New rules
			
			1. Don't draw blood if there is no ID band on the patient.
			
			2. The two officially recognized, hospital-wide patient identifiers are
			
			   • Patient's full name (first name, middle initial, and last name)
			
			   • Patient medical record number
			
			3. Place all computer labels beside, not on top of, any existing addressograph labels. (Note: This practice presents a challenge with pediatric specimen containers.)
			
			Next steps:
			
			1. Revise policy on specimen collection and labeling.
			
			2. Develop policy regarding two officially recognized patient identifiers.
			
			3. Add one more computer label printers in the emergency department (at opposite end of counter).
			
			4. Evaluate the appropriateness of placing computer label printers in ICU.
			
			5. Conduct an educational campaign.

Step 6: Test and carry out the redesigned processes

The team then pilot-tested each of these risk-reduction strategies to determine the impact that such a change in process would have on the other processes within the blood transfusion system.

Step 7: Measure the effectiveness of the redesigned process

Step 8: Maintain the effectiveness of the redesigned process over time

The final process improvements identified during the FMEA were then carried out facility-wide and transitioned into the organization's existing performance improvement process.

CHAPTER 2

RELATED ARTICLES

MISTAKES AND COMPLEXITY IN HEALTH CARE

Abstract

Hinckley and Barkan's conformance model predicts defect rates using three sources of defects: variance, mistakes, and complexity. Variance (and statistical process control) has been studied extensively generally and for health care. Mistakes and complexity have not been as widely addressed. This paper 1) presents evidence that demonstrates the importance of mistakes in health care processes, 2) discusses an approach to remediate mistakes, and 3) proposes an approach to assessing changes to a health care providers' process based on its relative priority and impact on complexity.

Introduction

In the late eighties and early nineties, many firms including health care organizations mounted substantial efforts to improve quality and customer satisfaction. These efforts centered on a corporate culture of employee empowerment and involvement, decision-making based on data, and statistical process control (SPC). More recently, many of these firms' efforts have been focused on documenting their processes in compliance with ISO 9000-based quality standards.

While these efforts have been important and effective in many cases, the framework for thinking about quality has been incomplete. This is particularly true when the definition of quality is the conformance- or manufacturing-based definition [Garvin 1988].

Hinckley and Barkan [1995] identify three sources of non-conformities, or defects: variance, mistakes, and complexity. Add to this the possibility of reducing defects through cultural means (incentives, awareness, driving out fear, etc.) [Hinckley 1997, Stewart & Grout 2001] and there are four distinct areas that must be addressed to achieve the single digit defects per million opportunities that are sought in today's highly competitive business environment. Of these only two are widely addressed in current quality practice: culture and variance. Variance as used here is the statistical variance that is usually managed using statistical tools like SPC, design of experiments, acceptance sampling, etc.

MISTAKES AND COMPLEXITY IN HEALTH CARE (CONT.)

Mistakes

Hinckley & Barkan [1995], and Chase & Stewart [1994] both argue that statistical variance based tools for controlling the process are not well suited to detecting mistakes caused by human error. Human error will often be classified as a common cause not a special cause. This is because human error tends to rare and intermittent. The impact of human errors on estimators of the process average and variance is likely to be small since they are likely to go undetected by sampling, or be discarded as an outlier. However, their impact is substantial when quality goals are in the range of single digit defects per million. Rook [1962] found that human errors in experimental settings are likely to reach nearly 300 defects per million for relatively simple operations. Leap [1994] found that errors are a much larger problem than that in the health care industry: approximately two percent (20,000 errors per million) of patient days involve an adverse drug reaction of some kind. McClelland, McMenamin, Moores, and Barbara [1996] report that individuals are 30 times more likely to die from human errors in the transfusion process than the more highly publicized risk of receiving HIV-tainted blood.

The approach to error prevention in health care (and elsewhere) has relied on individuals to not make errors [ABC news 1995, Small & Barach 2002 p. 1478]. The presumption has been that if errors occur, it indicates a lack of vigilance and determination by the individual. Similar approaches were, and often still are typical in industrial settings. The reflex among managers to exhort workers to "be more careful" is still common.

In quality management, it is often asserted that 85% of problems are attributable to "systems" outside the workers' control and that only 15% are attributable to workers. This has led managers to focus on improving systems instead of blaming workers for results that are out of their control. This approach is also appropriate for human errors. Donald Norman urges us to "change the attitude toward error. Think of an object's user as attempting to do a task, getting there by imperfect approximations. Don't think of the user as making errors; think of the actions as approximations of what is desired" [1989].

Methods for reducing mistakes and human error were developed at Toyota Motor Company by Shigeo Shingo [1986]. These methods make use of poka-yoke devices (pronounced POH-kah YOH-kay). Poka-yoke is Japanese for mistake-proofing. Poka-yoke devices are simple mechanisms that either prevent errors from occurring or make errors obvious before serious consequences result.

MISTAKES AND COMPLEXITY IN HEALTH CARE (CONT.)

Poka-yoke Framework

Poka-yoke devices have three attributes: an inspection method, a setting function, and a regulatory function. Each attribute is discussed in detail below.

Inspection methods. Shingo identified three types of inspection: judgment inspection, informative inspection, and source inspection. Judgment inspection sorts out defects. There is relative consensus that this type of inspection is discouraged.

Informative inspection is an inspection of the products produced by the process. Information from these product inspections is used as feedback to control the process and prevent defects. Control charts are one form of informative inspection. Shingo's successive checks and self-checks are alternative forms. These involve having each operation inspect the work of the prior operation, successive checks, or having workers assess the quality of their own work, self-checks. Informative inspections occur "after the fact."

Source inspection creates and uses feed-forward information to determine "before the fact" that conditions for error-free production exist. Norman [1989] refers to this type of device as a "forcing function" because these devices are often designed to prevent erroneous actions from occurring. Source inspection is preferred to informative inspection.

Source inspection, self-checks, and successive checks utilize 100% inspection of process outputs. These inspection techniques tend to increase the speed of quality feedback. Although every item is inspected, Shingo made it clear that inspection should lead to process improvements and prevent defects, and not merely sort out defects [Shingo, 1986, p. 57]. According to Shingo, source inspection is an ideal method of quality control because they insure that conditions for high quality production are assured before the process step is performed. Self-checks and successive checks may be used in those cases where source inspection cannot be done or when the cause and effect relationships of the process are not understood well enough to develop source inspections.

Setting Functions. A setting function is the method used to perform an inspection. Chase and Stewart [1995] identify four setting functions 1) physical 2) grouping and counting 3) sequencing and 4) infor-

MISTAKES AND COMPLEXITY IN HEALTH CARE (CONT.)

mation enhancement. Physical methods determine whether defects or problems exist based on the presence or absence of physical contact with a sensing device. The small bevel on one corner of 3.5-inch diskettes combined with a stop in the computer's disk drive eliminate the possibility of disks being inserted incorrectly into the computer. The grouping and counting method uses counting or measuring methods to insure no errors have occurred. Many firms uses product weight information and electronic scales to ensure that products or orders are complete and correct. Sequencing methods check that a standard sequence of actions occurs. In a car, the key must be switched on before the car is shifted out of park and must be shifted back to park before the keys can be removed. Information enhancement methods provide or preserve information that would not be available otherwise. Restaurants use pagers to allow patrons to stroll and shop without fear of not hearing that their table is ready.

Regulatory Functions. There are two regulatory functions: 1) warning functions and 2) control functions. The bells, buzzers, and warning lights in automobiles are warning functions. Their purpose is to warn that an error has occurred or is about to occur. Control functions are more restrictive than warning functions. They actually keep errors from occurring by stopping the process or in some cases correcting the process automatically. A car's gearshift mechanism is an example of a control function. The car cannot be shifted out of park unless the ignition key is inserted and turned to the on position. For more information on designing control functions, see Grout [2003].

Importance of mistake-proofing in health care

The fact that a patient is 30 times more likely to die as a result of a human error than to die from HIV tainted blood, along with the startling number of medication errors that occur in hospitals, indicates that mistake prevention is critical [IOM 1999].

To further demonstrate the importance of mistakes, consider the process of blood transfusions. After developing a flowchart for a blood transfusion process, numerous error modes were identified by doctors at the University of Texas Southwestern Medical school [Kaplan, 1995]. The majority of these errors can be grouped in to four categories (see Table 1 on the following page).

MISTAKES AND COMPLEXITY IN HEALTH CARE (CONT.)

Table 1

Error Category	Observations	Percentage of Items
Identifying & matching patients with their procedures and materials	13	23.2%
Information corruption through labeling, recording & data entry errors	14	25.0%
Insure availability of relevant information or information transfer	9	16.1%
Insure relevant information is used	4	7.1%
Other errors	16	28.6%
Total	56	100.0%

The errors in these four categories are human errors. They are unlikely to be common enough to be effectively managed using statistical descriptions of the variance. These categories can be characterized as identity-specific operations: patient-procedure-materials matching, moving information accurately through space and time, ensuring relevant information is available and used by service providers. The exercise of matching process steps with specific individuals and matching inputs with their uniquely acceptable recipient are pervasive throughout much of health care practice. Mistake-proofing these types of errors differs from the commonly implemented mistake-proofing devices identified in the literature [Shingo 1986, Nikkan Kogyo Shimbun 1988, Bayer 1994]. These mistakes are not however limited to health care. They also exist in business environment where traceability is important or where parts are not fully interchangeable, like some remanufacturing operations.

Medical applications examples

Templates have been used on a limited basis as part of the blood donation process. The templates are laid over patient forms so that improperly checked boxes and omitted data become more obvious.

MISTAKES AND COMPLEXITY IN HEALTH CARE (CONT.)

Surgeons use instrument trays with indentations for all of the instruments required in a procedure. The tray insures that all of the instruments are present. By replacing all instruments in the tray, a quick check can be made to insure all instruments are removed before closing the patient's incision.

The computer system at Brigham and Women's hospital that is used to process doctors' prescriptions [ABC News, 1995] is a mistake-proofing device. This is an example of computerized physician order entry (CPOE). Errors are reduced by allowing "point and click" selection of common dosages. The computer checks the prescription for possible overdoses (if manually entered), allergic reactions or reactions with other medicines the patient is taking. CPOE systems are being implemented in many hospitals, and drug store chains are using computerized systems to identify customers' drug interactions.

Blood-Loc is a combination-lock-secured disposable bag that is used to deliver a unit of blood to a specific patient. The combination for the lock is unique and only available to medical personnel on the patient's wrist ID. Blood-Loc insures that positive identification occurs before the blood can be unlocked and transfused. Burns and Wenz [1991] and AuBuchon [2001] provide a detailed description and indicate that specific erroneous transfusions were prevented by the Blood-Loc System.

Complexity

Hinckley and Barkan [1995] point out that complexity is also a source of non-conformities. They use design-for-assembly (DFA) techniques to measure complexity. This measure of complexity is correlated with the actual operation times in assembly processes [Hinckley, 1993]. He also shows that the DFA measure is also negatively correlated with non-conformities in industrial situations.

Reducing complexity essentially eliminates certain opportunities for errors to occur. Consider the experience of Weber Aircraft Operations. Weber Aircraft manufactures seats for passenger airliners. It had implemented numerous mistake-proofing devices to insure that the tubular aluminum frame of the seat was defect-free. In the mid-1990s, it started making some of these parts by milling a single piece of aluminum on a CNC machine. This process is preferred by DFA. The process costs less and avoids all the miss-cutting and welding process problems associated with tubular aluminum.

MISTAKES AND COMPLEXITY IN HEALTH CARE (CONT.)

In Motorola's quality program, the goal is 3.4 defects per million opportunities (DPMO). On any single product, there can be a large number of opportunities for defects to occur. The probability of producing a defect free product is the joint probability of all the opportunities being conforming. Reducing the opportunities for defects eliminates factors from the joint probability calculations. It is equivalent to insuring ongoing perfect quality for that opportunity.

Complexity in health care issues

Many of the process changes that occur in health care are the result of adverse outcomes and resulting corrective actions. Many of these corrective actions become changes to standard operating procedures (SOPs). As corrective actions are created and processed, the SOPs can be become very complicated. On occasion, the SOPs are so complicated that health care workers consciously circumvent the SOP using unapproved "work arounds." In many cases the complexity of the SOP is the cause of the workers' inability to comply with the SOP and the resulting adverse outcomes. Increased complexity of a procedure may increase the chance of error by making the basics of the process less obvious, thus increasing opportunities to commit error.

This suggests that changes to SOPs should be evaluated based on their impact on the system and on the criticality of the adverse effects of non-conformity. It is conceivable that SOPs are changed as part of a corrective action where the outcome is not severe and the occurrence of the non-conformity is rare. In such cases, the cost to the system from the added complexity may far outweigh the benefit from avoiding the outcome. As the number of modifications to the SOP increases, the complexity may increase exponentially rather than in a linear manner.

A preliminary analysis

In health care, indices of complexity like those used in DFA are yet to be developed. A specific complexity measure is not proposed here. Additional research in this area is needed. In the short term, the subjective predictions of time required to perform the process according to the SOP will be used as a measure of complexity. The DFA measures are refined means of predicting operation times. Those changes that increase the time required are considered to be more complex.

MISTAKES AND COMPLEXITY IN HEALTH CARE (CONT.)

The preliminary estimate of increased complexity must be compare with the relative priority number (RPN) of the adverse outcome. The concept of RPN comes from FMEA as presented by the Automotive Industry Action Group (AIAG) [1995]. In FMEA, the RPN is used to determine which failure modes deserve the most attention and where preventive measures should be focused first. FMEA allows many failure modes to be laid out on a worksheet and considered and prioritized simultaneously. Corrective action programs do not have this luxury. Corrective actions follow an arrival process where they must be considered serially. As a result, proper prioritization and measured responses are currently difficult to administer. Using the RPN along with a corresponding response policy would allow prioritization of the ongoing arrivals of corrective action requests. Often, responding to every corrective action request may only be possible if the response is a matter of expediency. Such expedient responses may make the system unduly complex or may not fully address the cause. The corrective action that states "the worker has been reprimanded and retrained" is common but not an effective corrective action. The admonition to "be more careful" is not effective since humans cannot obey over the long term.

The RPN is the product of three values: the criticality, the likelihood of occurrence, and the probability of detecting and remedying the non-conformance before any adverse effects can result. These three values are assessed subjectively along firm-specific guidelines. The values in the AIAG examples range from one to 10.

A Response policy that sets thresholds should be created by each firm over time to determine how to respond to various values of RPN. Cut off points like those shown in Table 2 can be established:

Table 2

RPN Rating	Response Level Required
RPN <250 & Criticality <3	No response
500>RPN>250	Minimal response
750>RPN>500	Respond w/o complexity increase
RPN>750	Immediate response followed by complexity reduction

MISTAKES AND COMPLEXITY IN HEALTH CARE (CONT.)

DeRosier et al [2002] provide a more qualitative response policy in their delineation of the health care FMEA process used by the Veteran's Administration. It uses the RPN concept but assigns descriptors rather than numeric values and then uses a decision tree to prescribe which failure modes need to be addressed.

The use of the RPN concept should have the effect of being an ongoing pareto-style analysis that determines which improvements should take priority. It allows this analysis to be done serially as the corrective actions are requested and allows a measured response to each event that occurs.

Many of the health care processes that have developed over time are tremendously complex. A lesson learned from SPC is that tampering with systems should be avoided. Even when a system is studied extensively, the bounded rationality of managers may result in situations where they make changes to the system for which the outcome is not completely understood. For very complex systems, managers may never be perfectly sure their changes are not tampering with the system. The use of RPN can provide an additional hurdle that changes must clear to avoid tampering.

Conclusions

Non-conformances in health care and elsewhere are the result of variance, mistakes, and complexity. The importance of mistakes in the context of health care has been demonstrated using data on a blood transfusion process and its potential failure modes. The applications of mistake-proofing or poka-yoke in health care applications has been presented along with examples. The management of complexity has been considered including a proposed tool for prioritizing corrective actions to avoid increasing complexity and making unwarranted changes to the system.

References

ABC News, 1995. "How to survive the hospital" 20/20 transcript #1527. Denver: Journal Graphics (July 7).

Aubuchon J: "Practical considerations in the implementation of measures to reduce mistransfusion.

MISTAKES AND COMPLEXITY IN HEALTH CARE (CONT.)

Transcript of Workshop on Best Practices for Reducing Transfusion Errors." Bethesda, MD: Food and Drug Administration, Feb 15, 2002, pp 74-94, 2002., *www.fda.gov/cber/minutes/0215bloo.pdf* (accessed on Jan 27, 2004).

Automotive Industry Action Group, 1995. "Process Failure Mode Effect Analysis."

Bayer, P.C. 1994. "Using Poka Yoke (Mistake Proofing Devices) to Ensure Quality." IEEE 9th Applied Power Electronics Conference Proceedings 1:201-204.

Chase, R.B., and D. M. Stewart. 1995. *Mistake-proofing: Designing Errors Out.* Portland, Oregon: Productivity Press.

Chase, R. B., and D. M. Stewart. 1994. "Make your service fail-safe." *Sloan Management Review* (Spring): 35-44.

DeRosier J, Stalhandske, E., Bagian, J.P., and Nudell, T. 2002. "Using health care failure mode and effect analysis: The VA National Center for Patient Safety's Prospective Risk Analysis System." *Joint Commission Journal on Quality Improvement* 28:248-267.

Garvin, David A. 1988. *Managing Quality: The Strategic and Competitive Edge.* New York: Free Press.

Grout J.R. 2003. "Preventing medical errors by designing benign failures." *Joint Commission Journal on Quality and Safety* 29(7): 354-362.

Hinckley, C.M. 1993. "A Global Conformance Quality Model: A New Strategic Tool for Minimizing Defects Caused by Variation, Error, and Complexity." (Dissertation) Ann Arbor Michigan: UMI Dissertation Services.

Hinckley, C.M. 1997. "Defining the best quality-control systems by design and inspection." *Clinical Chemistry* 43(5):873-879.

MISTAKES AND COMPLEXITY IN HEALTH CARE (CONT.)

Hinckley, C.M. and Barkan, P. 1995. "The role of variation, mistakes, and complexity in producing non-conformities." Journal of Quality Technology 27(3):242-249.

IOM: Committee on Quality of Health Care in America. Institutes of Medicine. 1999. *To Err is Human: Building a Safer Health System*. Washington, DC: National Academy Press.

Kaplan, H.S. 1995. personal communication and unpublished transfusion error mode data.

Leap, Lucian L. 1994. "Error in Medicine." *Journal of the American Medical Association* 272(23): 1851-1857.

McClelland, D.B.L., McMenamin, J.J., Moores, H.M., and Barbara, J.A.J. 1996. "Reducing risk in blood transfusion: process and outcome." *Transfusion Medicine* 6: 1-10.

Nikkan Kogyo Shimbun/Factory Magazine, (Ed.). 1988. *Poka-yoke: Improving product quality by preventing defects*. Portland, Oregon: Productivity Press.

Norman, D.A. 1989. *The Design of Everyday Things*. New York: Doubleday.

Rook, 1962. Sandia Labs report SCTM93-62(14).

Shingo, Shigeo. 1986. *Zero quality control: source inspection and the poka-yoke system*. trans. A.P. Dillion. Portland, Oregon: Productivity Press.

Small, S.D. and Barach, P. 2002. "Patient safety and health policy: a history and review." *Hematology/Oncology Clinics of North America* 16: 1463-1482.

Stewart, D.M. and Grout J.R. 2001. "The Human Side of Mistake-Proofing." *Production and Operations Management* 10(4):440-458.

Wenz, B. and Burns, E.R. 1991. "Improvement in transfusion safety using a new blood unit patient identification system as part of safe transfusion practice." *Transfusion*. 31 (5): 401-403.

Source: John R. Grout, www.mistakeproofing.com, *2004. Reprinted with permission.*

EXPERTS ANSWER QUESTIONS TO HELP IMPROVE YOUR **FMEA** PROCESS

Editor's note: We adapted these questions from the recent HCPro, Inc., audioconference, "FMEA Best Practices: Going beyond JCAHO compliance to improve patient safety." Experts Robert Marder, MD, and Craig Clapper spoke during the audioconference. HCPro publishes Briefings on Ambulatory Accreditation.

 Do we have to create a corrective action plan for every failure mode we identify as a result of the failure modes and effects analysis (FMEA)?

 Marder: No. Once you identify the failure modes, you determine the risk priority number (RPN). You should have a threshold number, and if something falls below that number, you don't need a corrective action.

Clapper: When people conduct an FMEA for the first time, they tend to have very high RPNs. The RPNs are based on the severity of the outcome of the error, how often the error is likely to occur, and how difficult it is to detect the error before it harms a patient.

When people are new to the FMEA process, they rate every error so it results in patient death every time, even though that is not realistic. In those cases, just develop corrective action plans for the top 10–25 failure modes.

 What is the difference between skill-based errors, knowledge-based errors, and rule-based errors?

 Marder: If you perform a routine task and make a mistake, this is a skill-based error. When thinking about what rule you need to follow at any given time, you can make a rule-based error in one of two ways. You can get the wrong information and then follow the wrong rule, or you know the rule but choose to ignore it. Knowledge-based errors occur when you attempt to do something you don't completely understand.

There is a one in 1,000 chance of making a skill-based error; a one in 100 chance of making a rule-based error, and a one in 10 chance of making a knowledge-based error.

Try to keep people from performing activities about which they have little knowledge.

EXPERTS ANSWER QUESTIONS TO HELP IMPROVE YOUR **FMEA** PROCESS (CONT.)

 How many people should participate in the FMEA process? Should the same people also complete the corrective action plans?

 Marder: There is no set number, but you want someone who is trained in and experienced with the FMEA process to guide people through the various steps. You also want a small group of professional experts from your staff who can provide examples of things that traditionally go wrong with certain procedures.

Try to have the FMEA committee meet three times: once to approve the process map and make sure the details are correct, another to identify various ways a procedure can fail, and the last to determine which corrective action plans to adopt based on the RPN numbers.

You don't want the process to take too much time, or it will be difficult to convince leaders to use an FMEA more frequently.

Source: Briefings on Ambulatory Accreditation, *August 2003, HCPro, Inc.*

Chapter 3

CASE STUDY:
MEDICATION USE FMEA

CHAPTER 3

Case Study: Medication Use FMEA

Medication errors are the fourth leading type of sentinel events, according to the Joint Commission on Accreditation of Healthcare Organizations (JCAHO) sentinel event database. The JCAHO reports on its Web site (*www.jcaho.org*) that medication errors account for nearly 12% of all sentinel events evaluated since it started reviewing such errors in 1995.

The National Coordinating Council for Medication Error Reporting and Prevention (NCC MERP) defines a medication error as "any preventable event that may cause or lead to inappropriate medication use or patient harm while the medication is in the control of the health care professional, patient, or consumer." Such events may be related to professional practice, health care products, procedures or systems (including prescribing;) order communication; product labeling, packaging, and nomenclature; compounding; dispensing; distribution; administration; education; monitoring; and use.[1]

National statistics on medication errors are alarming. In 2002, 482 health care organizations voluntarily reported 192,477 medication errors, according to MEDMARX, the national reporting database operated by the U.S. Pharmacopeia (USP), a nonprofit based in Rockville, MD. Although most of these errors never harmed the patient, 3,213 mistakes, or 1.7% of the total, did result in patient injury.

---

[1] *The NCC MERP Web site, www.nccmerg.org, 2003.*

Consider the following statistics:

Of the total 1.7% that resulted in patient injury

- 514 errors required some hospitalization
- 47 required life-sustaining interventions
- 20 (less than 1%) were fatal

The categories of drugs most commonly involved in errors were opioid analgesics, sedatives/hypnotics, and anticonvulsants. High-alert medications—including insulin, heparin, and morphine—were responsible for the most severe injuries. The top five errors reported (accounting for 88% of all types of errors) were

1. missed doses (one or more)
2. improper dose/quantity
3. prescribing error
4. wrong drug
5. wrong administration time

Incorrect administration techniques (when medications are incorrectly prepared or delivered, or both) were responsible for the largest number of harmful errors (6.2%).

In all, hospitals reported 54 causes of errors. The three causes typically involved in these errors included performance deficit, procedure or protocol not being followed, and communication errors across departments or disciplines. The USP has found that medication errors frequently result from distraction, increased workload, or use of temporary staff.

Looking at the JCAHO's retrospective review of sentinel events related to medication errors, orientation/training and communication account for approximately 60% and 55% of the root causes of these events, respectively.

Although technology such as computerized physician order entry (CPOE) and barcoding has been and will continue to be significant, an FMEA on the medication use process is a valuable exercise in helping organizations prioritize these and other less costly risk-reduction strategies.

Using the process outlined in Chapter 1, the following case study describes an FMEA on medication use. As with all FMEAs, the ultimate goal of this process is to reduce the risk of a devastating medication error occurring within an organization.

Step 1: Organize the team

Using the strategy explained in Chapter 1 to identify the most appropriate individuals to participate in an FMEA, the organization's leaders selected the following staff to serve on the team:

Core FMEA team members are as follows:

- Director, pharmacy
- Chief operating officer, facilitator
- Vice president, patient care services
- Clinical nurse manager, intensive care unit (ICU)
- Clinical nurse manager, step-down ICU
- Clinical nurse manager, emergency department
- Clinical nurse manager, medical/surgical unit
- Clinical nurse educator
- Information systems coordinator, nursing

Ad-hoc team members include:

- Clinical nurse manager, post anesthesia care
- Five unit secretaries
- Five registered nurses

Step 2: Flowchart the process

In a manner similar to the other case studies, using readily available software, the team flowcharted the medication use process. See Figure 3.1.

Step 3: Identify potential failure modes

The facilitator then led the FMEA team through a review of the finalized flowchart to identify steps in the process that might be vulnerable to break down. For example, when the practitioner writes the order, it could be illegible or a duplicate order, it may include the wrong choice of drug, route, or frequency. During the point in the process where the chart is flagged and placed in the rack, the flag may fall off or the chart may not be placed in the rack.

These, and other potential failure modes were then added to the flowchart (see the notations in Figure 3.1). For the sake of readability, not all of the failure modes that were identified by the FMEA team are affixed to the flowchart.

The potential failure modes were then entered into the matrix described in Chapter 1, and the group reached agreement on the frequency, severity, and detectability of the individual failure modes. From there, the team computed the risk priority number (RPN).

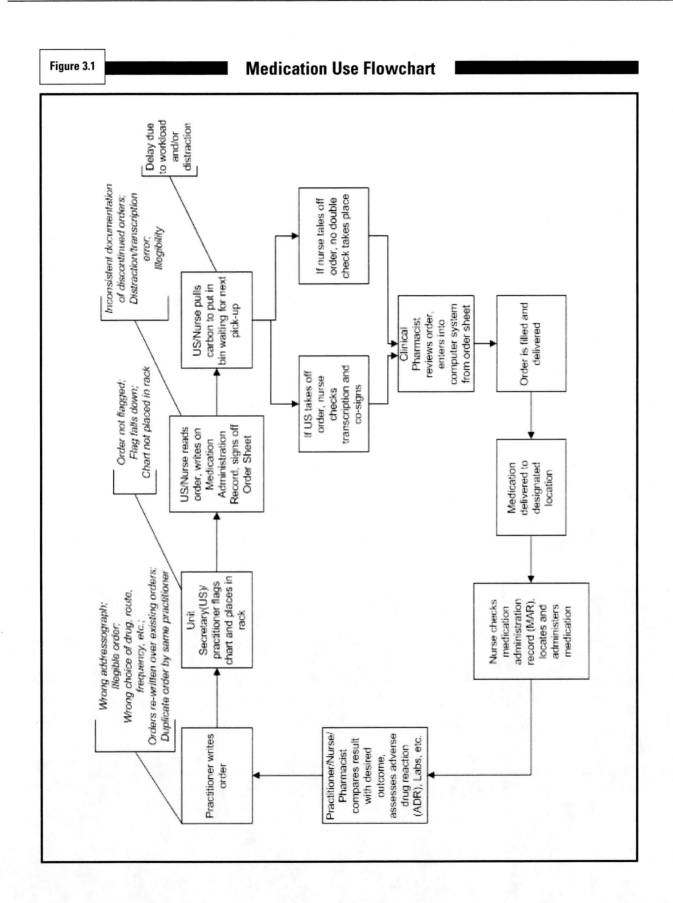

Figure 3.1   Medication Use Flowchart

Step 4: Identify the potential effect of each failure mode

For each potential failure mode, the team identified the ultimate impact on the patient. For instance, the team determined it is highly likely (a score of 10) that an illegible order could lead to a patient becoming severely harmed if a nurse or pharmacist misread the patient's name, drug, dose, route, or time. However, if it was decided that there would be a minor patient outcome (a score of 3) if one physician discontinues another's order and the patient missed a dose of medication.

This step resulted in the completed FMEA matrix, which appears in Figure 3.2. Unlike the coinciding matrices, which are sorted in decreasing order according to the RPN value, this matrix is organized in the order of the process, providing an alternative view of how RPNs may be displayed. This example allows anyone who reviews the FMEA to follow the logical flow of the process from beginning to end. It then might be helpful to sort the same matrix in descending order according to the RPN value.

Figure 3.2   **Medication Use RPN**

University Hospital and Medical Center
Failure Modes and Effects Analysis
Privileged and Confidential

Process to be assessed: Medication use (focusing on the ordering, transcribing, administration, and discontinuation stages of the process)

Potential failure mode	Potential effect of failure mode	Frequency (likeliness scale) 1–10	Severity (potential for harm) 1–10	Detectability (potential discovery) 1–10	Risk priority number (RPN)
Identify potential failures for each step in the process	Identify potential outcome of failure to patient	On a scale of 1–10 (10 = highly likely), identify the likelihood of this failure actually occurring Example: 1 = Remote probability 5 = Moderate probability 10 = Very high probability	On a scale of 1–10 (10 = worst potential failure outcome), identify the potential severity of the consequences of this failure. Example: 1 = Very minor outcome 5 = Moderate outcome 10 = Very severe outcome	On a scale of 1–10 (1 = failure easily discovered under normal circumstances highly likely), identify the potential difficulty of discovery of failure Example: 1 = Certain detection 5 = Possible detection 10 = Cannot detect	RPN = frequency X severity X detectability
Prescriber writes order					
Wrong addressograph	Wrong patient, wrong drug	3	10	5	150
Illegible order	Wrong patient, drug, dose, route or time	10	10	1	100
Prescriber writes order illegibly–over addressograph, on lines, too crowded	Missed order	7	10	1	70
Wrong choice of drugs, route or frequency	Delayed turn-around time or error	5	10	3	150
Orders not timed	Delayed turn-around time or missed dose	10	3	1	30
Orders re-written over existing orders - illegible	Wrong patient, drug, dose, route, or time	5	5	7	175
Duplicate order by same physician	Multiple doses administered, delayed turn-around time	2	6	4	48

Figure 3.2 — Medication Use RPN (cont.)

Process/Failure mode	Effect				RPN
Inconsistent use of generic v. brand name drug	Delayed turn-around time, wrong drug	10	10	7	700
One physician discontinues another's order(s)	Missed doses	3	3	1	9
Consultant → Attending or Attending → Covering attending					
Use of look-alike/sound-alike drugs	Wrong drug	4	10	8	320
Unit secretary (US)/ physician flags chart and places in rack:					
Order not flagged	Misses dose(s)	5	6	5	150
Flag fell down	Misses dose(s)	7	6	5	210
Chart not in rack	Misses dose(s)	7	6	5	210
US/nurse reads order, writes on medication administration record (MAR), signs off order sheet:					
Inconsistent documentation of discontinued orders	Too many dose(s)	9	10	1	90
Inconsistency with who transcribes orders— inconsistent role/use of US: some transcribe all orders onto MAR, some transcribe none.	No immediate impact	10	5	4	200
Distraction	Missed dose(s), wrong patient, drug, dose, route, or time	10	10	4	400
Illegibility	Delays, wrong patient, drug, dose, route, or time	5	5	1	25
No transcription of order to MAR	Missed dose(s)	5	10	5	250
Chart misplaced	Missed dose(s)	6	6	1	36
Error in transcription	Delays, wrong patient, drug, dose, route, or time	3	10	5	150
Discontinued orders not sent to Pharmacy	Too many dose(s)	8	5	2	80
Faxed orders not legible	Delays, missed dose(s)	8	10	8	640

Figure 3.2 — **Medication Use RPN (cont.)**

US/nurse pulls carbon to put in pharmacy bin waiting for pick-up					
Delay due to workload or distraction	Delays, missed dose(s)	9	6	4	216
Order sits in bin until hourly pharmacy rounds	Delays, missed dose(s)	6	6	1	36
If US takes off orders – nurse checks and co-signs; If nurse takes off order—no check takes place:					
Transcription error	Delays, wrong patient, drug, dose, route, or time	3	10	4	120
No allergies	Allergic reaction	2	2	1	4
No patient weight or height	Delay in order processing	2	10	5	100
Nurse checks MAR, locates meds, administers meds:					
Meds not transferred with patient by care provider	Delay in order processing, missed dose(s)	9	6	1	54
Nurse looks in wrong location for meds (e.g., refrigerator, drawer, or counter.)	Delay in order processing, missed dose(s)	6	5	1	30
24-hour chart heck to verify that all orders were transcribed and compare MAR and orders to ensure that all orders were appropriately carried out:					
24-hour chart check not completed accurately	Missed dose(s), wrong patient, drug, dose, route, or time	3	8	5	120
	Missed dose(s)	4	4	4	64

Step 5: Redesign the processes/underlying systems

The team then held a session to brainstorm potential improvements to the existing processes to reduce the risk of their breaking down and having the identified impact on the patient. For example, to reduce the inconsistent use of a generic or brand name drug, the team established the following two-step process:

- The director of pharmacy services will print out the formulary/drug list to include the brand name, generic name, pharmacologic category, dose/strength, and dosage form. The list is then placed in a binder, which is attached to each medication cart.

- The director of pharmacy services will also address the ordering practices of the prescriber. The pharmacy must require prescribers to write medication orders using generic and brand names and be consistent in the use of those names. The director is also required to present the issue to the medical staff through the pharmacy and therapeutics committees and medical executive committee.

See Figure 3.3. for the complete results of this brainstorming activity.

Step 6: Test and implement the redesigned process(es)

The team then pilot-tested each of the risk-reduction strategies to determine the impact that such a change in process would have on the other processes within the system of medication use.

Step 7: Measure the effectiveness of the redesigned process

Step 8: Maintain the effectiveness of the redesigned process over time

The final process improvements emanating FMEA were then carried out facility-wide and transitioned into the organization's existing performance improvement process.

<table>
<tr><td>Figure 3.3</td><td colspan="2">**Medication Use Risk-Reduction Efforts**</td></tr>
</table>

University Hospital and Medical Center
Failure Modes and Effects Analysis
Privileged and Confidential

Process to be addressed: Medication Use

Potential failure mode	Responsible party	Risk priority number (RPN)	Process improvement/ risk reduction effort
Inconsistent use of generic v. brand name drug	1. Director, pharmacy services	700	1. Print out formulary/drug list to include brand name, generic name, pharmacologic category, dose/strength, and dosage form (cross-referenced: Brand → Generic; by pharmacologic category; and Generic → Brand); place in sleeves/ binders; and chain to each medication cart/medication room.
	2. Director, pharmacy services		2. Address the ordering practices of prescriber— "require" prescribers to write medication orders using generic and brand names—or within a single order; have the prescriber be consistent (using brand or generic names consistently). Present issue to medical staff (through pharmacy and therapeutics committee (P&T) and medical executive committee).
Faxed orders not legible	1. Director, pharmacy services	640	1. Install fax machine system with memory bank. (System works as follows: Pharmacy pulls up orders on image-enhanced screen, system triages orders—unit-specific, STAT v. non-STAT).

Figure 3.3 **Medication Use Risk-Reduction Efforts (cont.)**

Distraction Inconsistency with who transcribes orders. Inconsistent role/use of unit secretary (Some transcribe all orders onto medication admin-istration record (MAR), some transcribe none.)	1. Vice president (VP), patient care services 2. VP, patient care services 3. VP, patient care services	400 260	1. Unit secretaries will consistently transcribe all orders. 2. Organize "in" and "out" baskets of charts with orders "to be transcribed" and "orders already transcribed." 3. Structure/standardize the workflow of unit secretaries.
Use of look-alike/ sound-alike drugs	P&T committee	320	Review and revise formulary
No transcription of order to MAR Inconsistent documentation of discontinued orders Missed dose(s)	1. VP, patient care services a. VP, patient care services b. Director, nursing education 2. VP, patient care services 3. VP, patient care services	250 270 270	1. In order to reduce transcription errors and missed medications, the unit secretary will transcribe **all** orders (medication and non-medication). a. Revise/reinforce unit secretary job description accordingly. b. Provide medical terminology training to existing unit secretaries and incorporate into orientation program. 2. Upon patient transfer from one unit to another, nurses will write "transfer to 851A," summarize the orders (otherwise the medication will be delivered to the unit that the patient was transferred *from*), and re-do the med sheet. 3. Initiate 24-hour chart checks (on the night shift), with the clinical manager assigning

Figure 3.3 ■■■■ **Medication Use Risk-Reduction Efforts (cont.)** ■■■■

			responsibility to a specific individual and assuring that they are completed.
	4. VP, patient care services		4. When the nurse leaves the floor, they are to notify the unit secretary and place the red binder in the rack at the desk.
	5. Chief medical officer		5. Implement more widespread use of pre-printed orders.
	6. Director, pharmacy services/VP, patient care services (with medical staff approval)		6. Change the design of the MAR **and** the narcotic sheet. a. Decide on redesign b. Draft policies and procedures regarding MAR sheets for consistent use and how to complete sheets c. Educate staff regarding policy d. Implement redesign
Nurse looks in wrong location for meds (e.g., refrigerator, drawer, counter.) Medications in nurse servers are from a previous patient's stay, leading to confusion and administration of wrong medication	1. Director, pharmacy services/ clinical managers		1. Purchase and implement use of standardized medication carts. a. Clinical managers to confirm their needs (# of carts) b. Order carts c. Implement use

CHAPTER 3

RELATED ARTICLES

AUTOMATED SYSTEM ENSURES ACCURACY

Using a computerized physician order entry (CPOE) system helped one New England facility reduce errors, comply with medication standards, and direct its focus to patient care.

The Joint Commission on Accreditation of Healthcare Organizations' (JCAHO) medication standard MM.4.10 requires organizations to review all prescriptions to ensure the appropriateness of the drug, dose, and frequency. The JCAHO also requires a pharmacist to review all medication orders unless a delay would harm the patient.

The 606-bed Maine Medical Center in Portland, ME, has used CPOE for more than 20 years, and recently upgraded its system in July to include medication alerts and a standardized nationwide database of drug interactions, says Miriam Leonard, RPh, MS, vice president of operations and patient safety officer.

How the system works

The new CPOE system uses the Multum database, which alerts a physician to any possible drug interactions that could occur and provides alternative medications.

A physician can override the alert, but he or she must acknowledge that the alert occurred, Leonard says. A pharmacist can also receive the alert, allowing him or her to question the physician about the prescription.

The physician logs onto the CPOE system and selects the medication, chooses the medication strength, adds any instructions, and sends it to the pharmacy.

Physicians can also log onto Maine Medical Center's system from their homes or offices.

The pharmacist reviews the order, checks for allergies and other side effects, and then processes the order. For unit-dose prescriptions, a robotic arm then picks out the drugs based on a package code and fills the order. Pharmacists still fill intravenous medication orders manually, Leonard says.

AUTOMATED SYSTEM ENSURES ACCURACY (CONT.)

Reducing confusion

The automated system reduces questions about similar-sounding or similar-looking medications and illegible handwriting, Leonard says. Staff members can spend more time focusing on the patient's treatment than on correcting medication errors.

"It takes away a lot of the problems of interpretation," she says.

TIP: Clarify any questions about the medication with the physician prior to filling the order.

The hospital maintains a policy for emergency situations, Leonard says. Authorized nurse practitioners or physician's assistants can enter orders into the system in some cases. A pharmacist would still have to review the order later.

The hospital stores some medications on the floor for emergency use, and the pharmacy has a "stat pager" that allows staff to call in orders from care areas in an urgent situation.

Pharmacy employees run some medications to physicians, while pharmacists can rush other medications to areas of the hospital through a network of tubes similar to those at bank drive-up windows.

Handling after-hours access

Maine Medical Center's pharmacy is open 24 hours a day, so after-hour access issues do not arise, Leonard says. A pharmacist is always on duty.

TIP: If you don't have a pharmacy that is always open, create a process that allows a pharmacist to review emergency and after-hours orders.

For example, the pharmacist reviews the order as soon as he or she is available after the emergency or as soon as the pharmacy opens.

AUTOMATED SYSTEM ENSURES ACCURACY (CONT.)

Any error detection system requires staff education. Medication administration is primarily the nursing staff's responsibility, so Maine Medical Center ensures that all new nurses receive comprehensive training in their orientation, Leonard says.

For example, nurses in the oncology department must be aware of chemotherapy standards and medications used in that specialty, in addition to general medication administration practices.

Nurses must also undergo annual competency training and skills updates, she says.

Train staff annually

Physicians must receive continuing education on an annual basis as well. The physician's professional organization and the hospital both participate in that education, which consists of a number of hours determined by the professional group and hospital requirements, Leonard says.

Education is also a priority when a hospital puts a new medication error detection system in place. Staff members must become oriented with state, federal, and accreditation requirements and standards as well as the system's operating procedures.

Maine Medical Center created online training for its new CPOE system, allowing physicians to learn how to enter orders and pharmacists to verify and fill them, Leonard says.

Source: Hospital Pharmacy Regulation Report, *October 2003, published by HCPro, Inc.*

MEDICATION ERROR REPORT FOCUSES ON JCAHO GOALS

Tips for pharmacists to reduce errors, improve safety

The pressure is on to clamp down on how you handle high-alert medications. In fact, the Joint Commission on Accreditation of Healthcare Organizations (JCAHO) in 2004 will score how you fare in this area.

Four of the JCAHO's seven National Patient Safety Goals cover medication administration, says Rod Hicks, RN, MSN, MPA, research coordinator for the U.S. Pharmacopeia's (USP) Center for the Advancement of Patient Safety (CAPS) and co-author of the Summary of Information Submitted to MEDMARX in the Year 2002: The Quest for Quality, released November 18, 2003. The goals relating to medication include the following:

- Improve high-alert medication safety
- Improve the accuracy of patient identification
- Improve communication among caregivers
- Improve the safety of infusion pumps

High-alert medications such as insulin, morphine, heparin, and potassium chloride represented 35.1% of the cases resulting in patient harm in 2002, according to the report. USP researchers also focused on errors in the geriatric population. Miscommunication and misidentification were harmful to elderly patients, with 55% of all fatal hospital medication errors involving seniors.

USP oversees MEDMARX, an anonymous Internet medication error reporting database. Researchers noticed reported errors increased to 192,477 in 2002, up from 105,603 in 2001. According to the report, 3,213 errors (1.7%) resulted in patient harm in 2002, compared to 2.4% in 2001.

This is due to more hospitals subscribing to MEDMARX—482 in 2002 compared to 368 in 2001—and better internal error reporting procedures, Hicks says. USP charges hospitals a fee based on their number of beds to join MEDMARX, Hicks says. USP uses the money to fund the MEDMARX program.

"There's more awareness to report errors," Hicks says. "We want all errors reported, whether they involve harm or not."

MEDICATION ERROR REPORT FOCUSES ON JCAHO GOALS (CONT.)

Pay attention to high-alert meds

Eight of the top 10 products causing harm to the patient in 2002 were high-alert medications, drugs more likely to cause an adverse reaction if given improperly. These medications include insulin, morphine, heparin, potassium chloride, warfarin, hydromorphone, fentanyl, and meperidine.

Of the high-alert medications, insulin errors resulted in patient harm 8.1% of the time. One reason is that one larger teaching hospital had as many as 27 different scales for insulin dosing, Hicks says. In fact, he adds, each unit may have a different dosing scale.

TIP: Standardize insulin dosing at your hospital.

There are more than 20 different formulations of insulin, according to Hicks. For example, intermediate formulations last for up to 24 hours in the patient, whereas short duration could last a few hours, he says.

When the pharmacy sends insulin vials to the floor, staff sometimes place vials in boxes labeled "regular" or "intermediate," depending on the dose of the vials in the box, Hicks says. The problem, Hicks explains, is that sometimes vials get placed in the wrong box. Staff do not look at the vials before administering them to patients, giving the wrong dose in the process.

TIP: Look at the vial's label instead of relying on the box label.

"It's not a high-tech solution," Hicks says. "Just throw the outer container away."

Double-check for safety

Hicks suggests that pharmacists be careful with patient weight. Conversions between pounds and kilograms often troubles physicians, pharmacists, and nurses, he says. For example, heparin doses depend on the patient's weight. If a physician writes the order in kilograms and the weight must be converted from pounds, the potential for error exists because someone may not do the math correctly.

TIP: Use laminated cards that convert kilograms to pounds. Double-check the conversion before filling the order.

ID the correct patient

Computers systems may also cause patient identification problems. Computer entry was the fourth overall cause of errors in 2002, with 17,998 errors recorded. It was seventh overall in 2000 and fifth in 2001, Hicks says.

System design is one reason for errors, Hicks says. For example, a prescriber may confuse James Brown Sr. with James Brown Jr. because there is no distinction between each row on the computer screen.

"What's happening visually is the prescriber is seeing one name on the screen, but the eye doesn't follow to that suffix," Hicks says. "You need to make each line discernable by highlighting every other one."

TIP: Design computer entry systems that highlight every other line or prohibit physicians from prescribing medications for patients other than their own.

Keep track of seniors' meds

Communication is a major issue when dealing with senior citizens, Hicks says. Seniors often see multiple specialists or pass through more than one department while in a hospital. For example, an elderly patient could move from the ER to internal medicine to the cardiac unit, with physicians prescribing medications in each department.

Physicians could prescribe contradictory therapies or staff could misplace medication orders when a patient moves from one unit to another, Hicks says. To avoid this, patients should carry a list of their medications wherever they go. This will help hospital staff avoid giving a drug that could interact with medication the patient already takes.

MEDICATION ERROR REPORT FOCUSES ON JCAHO GOALS (CONT.)

Beware of infusion pumps

The JCAHO wants facilities to use infusion pumps that avoid free, or uncontrolled, flow of the solution, Hicks says. Facilities should also focus on programming the pumps correctly to ensure the patient receives the proper dose.

USP researchers found 1,846 errors involving an infusion pump, 161 of which caused patient harm. Staff often programmed the pumps wrong, giving the patient too much or too little of a medication.

For example, a 60-year-old patient had an order for an initial meperidine dose of 20 mg followed by 10 mg every 12 minutes, not to exceed 180 mg in four hours. The patient became unresponsive after receiving an initial 170-mg dose instead because a staff member programmed the pump wrong, according to the report.

TIP: Clearly label IV bags with the patient name, medication, dosage, and infusion rate.

Hospitals could consider smart IV pumps, which allow hospitals to program minimum and maximum dosage ranges for medications, Hicks says. Staff would receive a warning if they entered a dose outside of the accepted range.

Editor's note: For more information on the MEDMARX survey, go to www.usp.org.

Source: Hospital Pharmacy Regulation Report, February 2004, published by HCPro, Inc.

QUICK FIXES WON'T SOLVE MEDICATION SYSTEM PROBLEMS

Don't use quick solutions—such as sending out memos or using extra warning labels—to fix problems with your medication system, according to Glenn Krasker, MHSA, president of Critical Management Solutions, a consulting firm based in Wilmington, DE.

During a recent audioconference titled, "Medication Management: How to Use FMEA to Identify High Risk Areas in your System, Krasker and other experts offered failure modes and effects analysis (FMEA) strategies and tips to help you put in place improvements that will stick.

Make high-impact changes

JCAHO medication standard MM.8.10 requires organizations to evaluate their medication management systems for risk points. Conducting an FMEA is one way to do that. You need a high-impact solution to make the changes effective, Krasker said. Some high-impact solutions include the following:

- Simplifying medication administration processes and removing unnecessary steps

- Engineering controls, such as an intravenous tubing lock or bar coding

- Getting leadership involved in planning and instituting medication safety reforms

"Often, low-impact solutions are the only actions [facilities] take," said John Santell, MS, RPh, director of educational program initiatives at U.S. Pharmacopeia's Center for the Advancement of Patient Safety. "It's better to balance a total set of actions."

TIP: Combine sending out memos and using new warning labels with a policy change and the support of senior leadership, Krasker says.

QUICK FIXES WON'T SOLVE MEDICATION SYSTEM PROBLEMS (CONT.)

Identify the risks

If your organization focuses an FMEA on prescribing aspects, such as wrong doses or wrong drugs, you should form a committee to evaluate the process. Ask the following questions when identifying risks in the process:

- Who performs each task in the process we are evaluating?
- What could go wrong?
- What is the possible impact on the patient?

Use a flow chart to outline the process and identify risky activities, Krasker said. He recalled one situation in which a prescriber ordered a medication that resulted in a harmful interaction with the Coumadin the patient was already taking. The patient had an adverse reaction and had to stay in the hospital five extra days. When the team examined the process, they noticed that the prescriber was unfamiliar with the potential interaction.

A solution to this problem would be to circulate a list of drugs that adversely interact with commonly prescribed drugs such as Coumadin.

Source: Briefings on Ambulatory Accreditation, *January 2004, HCPro, Inc.*

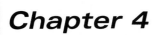

Chapter 4

CASE STUDY: PATIENT SUICIDE FMEA

CHAPTER 4

Case Study: Patient Suicide FMEA

Patient suicide ranks as the number-one type of sentinel event reviewed by the Joint Commission on Accreditation of Healthcare Organizations (JCAHO) since it began evaluating such errors in 1995.

Although patient suicide is by far most pervasive in psychiatric hospitals, nonhospital behavioral health care settings, and psychiatric units in general hospitals, it also occurs in general hospital emergency departments and in long-term care facilities.

According to the JCAHO's retrospective review of this type of sentinel event, the physical environment and patient assessment process represent the most common root causes. This sheds light onto areas where an organization might focus its patient suicide FMEA.

It's easy to alter the physical environment in the units/areas in which high-risk patient populations receive care (e.g., psychiatric units) to reduce the potential for suicide. But it's impractical to undertake such alterations throughout a general, acute care hospital. Thus, the following FMEA case study shows that organizations might place more attention on the patient assessment process and appropriate patient placement to reduce the risk of patient suicide. As with all FMEAs, the ultimate goal of this exercise is to reduce the risk of patients harming themselves through their interaction with the environment.

Step 1: Organize the team

Using the strategy explained in Chapter 1, the organization's leaders selected the following staff to serve on the team:

Core team members:

- Director of nursing
- Risk manager, facilitator
- Two behavioral health technicians
- Director of physical plant operations
- Biomedical engineer
- Director, environmental services
- Clinical nurse manager, emergency department
- Clinical nurse manager, medical/surgical units
- Chief of psychiatry
- Nurse educator
- Safety officer

Ad-hoc team members:

- Four registered nurses
- Two nursing assistants

Step 2: Flowchart the process

In a manner similar to the other case studies, using readily available software, the team flowcharted the medication use process, which appears in Figure 4.1.

Figure 4.1

Figure 4.1 — Patient Suicide Flowchart

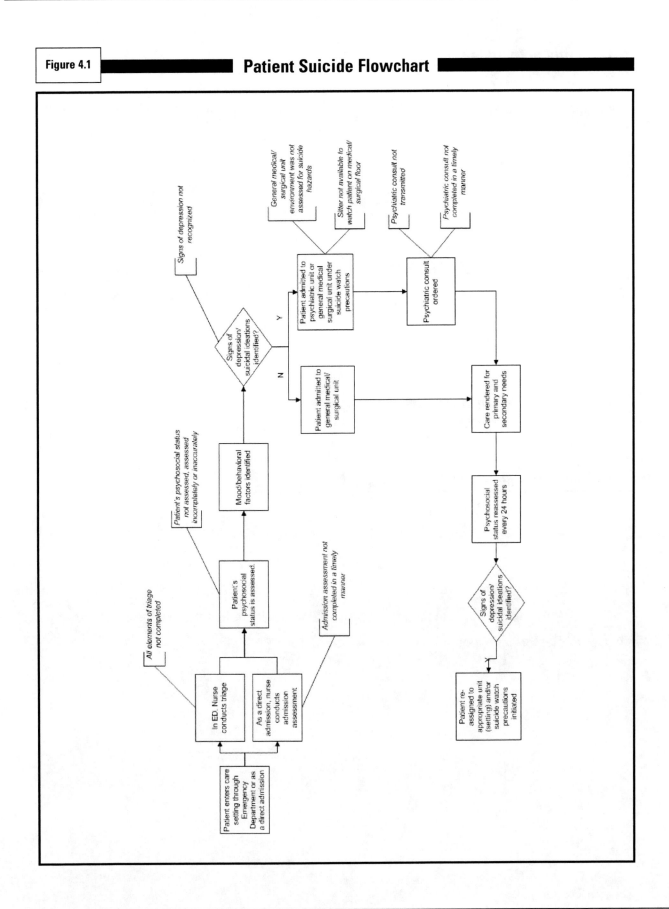

Step 3: Identify potential failure modes

Continuing the process outlined in Chapter 1, the facilitator then led the FMEA team through a review of the finalized flowchart to identify individual steps in the process that might be vulnerable to break down. For example, a patient is admitted to a general medical/surgical unit under suicide watch precautions. This step in the process could break down if that unit environment wasn't assessed for suicide hazards or if a sitter wasn't available to watch the patient on the medical/surgical floor.

The team added this and other potential failure modes to the flowchart. (See the sampling identified in brackets in Figure 4.1. For readability, not all of the failure modes identified by the FMEA team are affixed to the flowchart.)

The team then entered the potential failure modes into the matrix described in Chapter 1, and the group reached agreement on the frequency, severity, and detectability of the individual failure modes. This process allowed the team to compute the risk priority number (RPN).

Step 4: Identify the potential effect of each failure mode

For each of the potential failure modes, the team identified the ultimate impact on the patient. For example, if the general medical/surgical unit environment wasn't assessed for suicide hazards, it's possible that the patient could be seriously hurt (a score of 10) using the equipment/supplies in the area. See Figure 4.2 for the completed FMEA matrix, which identifies the likeliness of the event occurring, potential for harm, potential discoverability, and the RPN.

Figure 4.2 ■ **Patient Suicide RPN** ■

General Hospital
Failure Modes and Effects Analysis
Privileged and Confidential

Process to be assessed: Patient suicide

Potential failure mode	Potential effect of failure mode	Frequency (likeliness scale) 1–10	Severity (potential for harm) 1–10	Detectability (potential discovery) 1–10	Risk priority number
Triage assessment incomplete	Signs of depression/suicide not recognized.	2	10	5	100
Admission assessment not completed in a timely manner	Signs of depression/suicide not recognized early enough in patient's stay.	2	10	5	100
Patient's psychosocial status not assessed, assessed incompletely, or assessed inaccurately	Signs of depression/suicide not recognized.	3	10	9	270
Failure in the assessment process to identify signs of depression/suicidal ideations.	Signs of depression/suicide not recognized.	4	10	8	320
The importance of stress, recent losses, unemployment, and response to stress (e.g., excess sleeping) not noted as signs of depression and acted upon.	Signs of depression/suicide not recognized.	3	9	10	270

Figure 4.2 ■ Patient Suicide RPN (cont.) ■

Patient not assigned to appropriate unit to provide adequate observation for signs of suicide.	Patients can harm themselves with the physical environment, equipment/supplies.	3	10	9	270
General medical/surgical unit environment was not assessed for suicide hazards.	Patients can harm themselves with the physical environment, equipment/supplies.	3	10	5	150
Sitter not available to watch patients on medical/surgical floor.	Patients' behaviors leading up to self-inflicted harm not identified.	2	8	1	16
Psychiatric consult not transmitted.	Suicidal ideations not identified.	1	10	5	50
Psychiatric consult not completed in a timely manner.	Suicidal ideations not identified in a timely manner.	2	10	1	20

Step 5: Redesign the processes/underlying systems

The next step was to brainstorm potential improvements to the existing processes to reduce the risk of their breaking down and having the identified impact on the patient. For example, the team identified a potential failure mode as the failure in the assessment process to identify signs of depression or suicidal thoughts. During the brainstorming session, the team outlined the following plan to reduce the risk of this failure mode occurring:

- The nursing educator will make sure that nursing and medical staff members will receive the following inservice education:
    - Recognizing the signs and symptoms of depression
    - Conducting a nursing assessment of the depressed patient (including frequency of reassessment)
    - Recognizing depression in the medical setting
    - Assessing for suicidal tendencies

- Develop a checklist that includes the signs and symptoms for depression (prompts of what to look for) and a scale to measure the patient's risk of suicide.

See Figure 4.3 for the risk-reduction efforts for each of the potential failure modes.

Figure 4.3 **Patient Suicide Risk-Reduction Efforts**

General Hospital

Failure Modes and Effects Analysis

Privileged and Confidential

Process to be assessed: Patient suicide

Potential failure mode	Responsible party	Risk priority number	Process improvement/risk reduction effort
Patient's psychosocial status not assessed, assessed incompletely, or assessed inaccurately	Director of nursing	270	Incorporate evaluation of psychosocial assessment into daily chart checks to verify that patient's psychosocial assessment is completed.
Failure in the assessment process to identify signs of depression/ suicidal ideations	Nursing educator	270	Nursing and medical staff members will receive inservice education on • recognizing the signs and symptoms of depression • conducting a nursing assessment of the depressed patient (including frequency of reassessment) • recognizing depression in the medical setting • assessing for suicide ideations Develop a checklist of signs and symptoms for depression (prompts of what to look for) and a scale to measure the patient's risk of suicide.
The importance of stress, recent losses, unemployment, and response to	Chief of psychiatry	270	Develop a standing protocol reflecting that any patient meeting a predefined threshold for depression and risk of

Figure 4.3

Patient Suicide Risk-Reduction Efforts (cont.)

stress (e.g., excess sleeping) not noted as signs of depression and acted upon			suicide will automatically trigger a consult by the psychiatrist.
Patient not assigned to appropriate unit to provide adequate observation for signs of suicide	Chief of psychiatry	270	Based upon the psychiatrist's assessment, determine whether the patient needs to be transferred to the behavioral health unit.
	Safety officer		Conduct a hazard analysis to identify factors that could be used by patients at risk for suicide.
	Chief of psychiatry		Develop criteria for transfer to a behavioral health unit.

Step 6: Test and implement the redesigned process(es)

The team then pilot-tested each risk-reduction strategy to determine the impact that such a change in process would have on the other processes associated with reducing the risk of patient suicide.

Step 7: Measure the effectiveness of the redesigned process

Step 8: Maintain the effectiveness of the redesigned process over time

The final process improvements identified throughout the patient suicide FMEA were then carried out facility-wide and transitioned into the organization's existing performance improvement processes.

Chapter 5

CASE STUDY:
WRONG-SITE SURGERY FMEA

CHAPTER 5

Case Study: Wrong-Site Surgery FMEA

Although there have been many widely publicized medical errors over the years, perhaps the initial case that caught the health care industry and the public's attention involved Willie King, a man from Florida whose wrong leg was reportedly amputated. This case was the first of many to be reported in the media and initiated many state governments and the Joint Commission on Accreditation of Healthcare Organizations (JCAHO) to develop a formal response to such sentinel events.

The American Academy of Orthopaedic Surgeons (AAOS) has identified wrong-site surgery as a devastating problem that affects both the patient and surgeon. It is not just an error that occurs because the surgeon operates on the wrong limb. Rather, the AAOS has determined that it is a systems problem that originates from the following actions:

- Poor preoperative planning
- Lack of institutional controls
- Failure of the surgeon to exercise due care
- A breakdown in communication between the surgeon and the patient or staff

The JCAHO has identified wrong-site surgery as the third leading type of sentinel event experienced by accredited organizations since the JCAHO first started reviewing such errors in 1995[1]. The JCAHO database reflects that wrong-site surgery accounted for more than 12% of all sentinel events it has reviewed.

[1] *Sentinel event statistics, JCAHO Web site, www.jcaho.org, 2004.*

The problem of wrong-site surgery is so significant that the JCAHO published two *Sentinel Event Alerts* on the topic, targeted the issue with a National Patient Safety Goal, and approved the Universal Protocol for Preventing Wrong Site, Wrong Procedure and Wrong Person Surgery™.

The JCAHO established the universal protocol because wrong-site surgeries continue despite national attention and efforts by professional associations and regulatory groups. This protocol consists of specific processes organizations must follow during preoperative verification, site-marking of the operative site, and the "time out" immediately before starting the procedure. In an effort to reduce the incidence of these tragic medical errors, the JCAHO requires all accredited hospitals, ambulatory care, and office-based surgery facilities to comply with the universal protocol effective July 1, 2004.

As the preoperative preparation process involves a significant number of hand-offs among staff from multiple units or areas, it should come as no surprise that nearly 8% of the sentinel events relating to wrong-site surgery reviewed by the JCAHO identified communication as a root cause.

The importance of creating systems and processes that formalize communication will be evident through the following case study. As with all FMEAs, the ultimate goal of this FMEA is to reduce the risk of wrong-site surgery occurring within an organization.

Step 1: Organize the team

Using the strategy explained in Chapter 1, the organization's leaders selected the following staff to serve on the FMEA teams:

Core team members:

- Clinical manager, operating room (OR)
- Vice president, patient care services, facilitator
- Supervisor, preoperative holding
- OR circulating nurse
- OR scrub nurse

- Chief of anesthesia
- Chief of surgery
- Orthopaedic surgeon
- Clinical nurse manager, med/surg unit

Ad-hoc team members include:

- Two medical surgical registered nurses

Step 2: Flowchart the process

In a manner similar to the other case studies, using readily available software, the team flowcharted the presurgical process, which appears in Figure 5.1 on the following pages.

Figure 5.1

Wrong-Site Surgery Flowchart

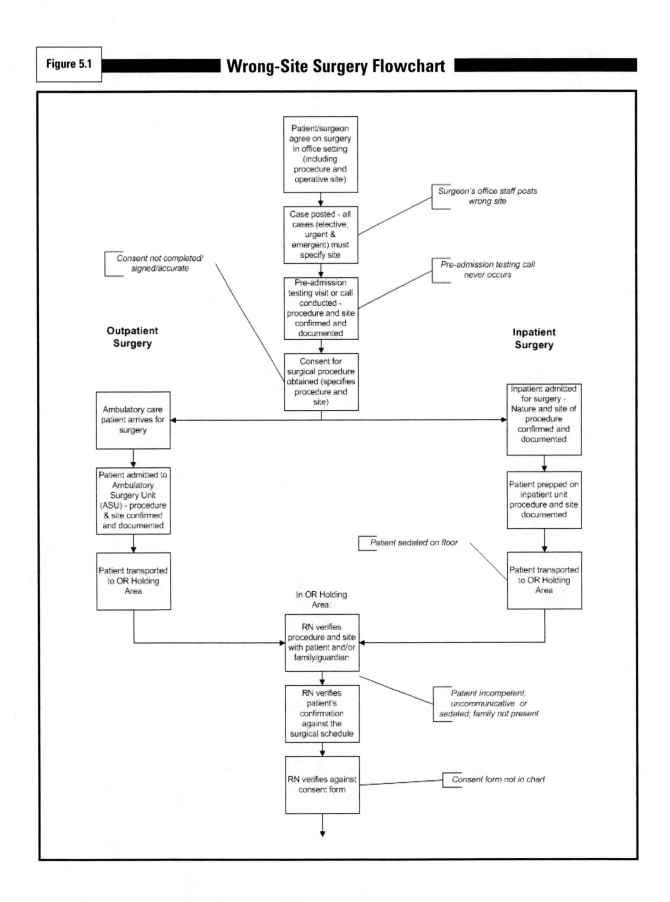

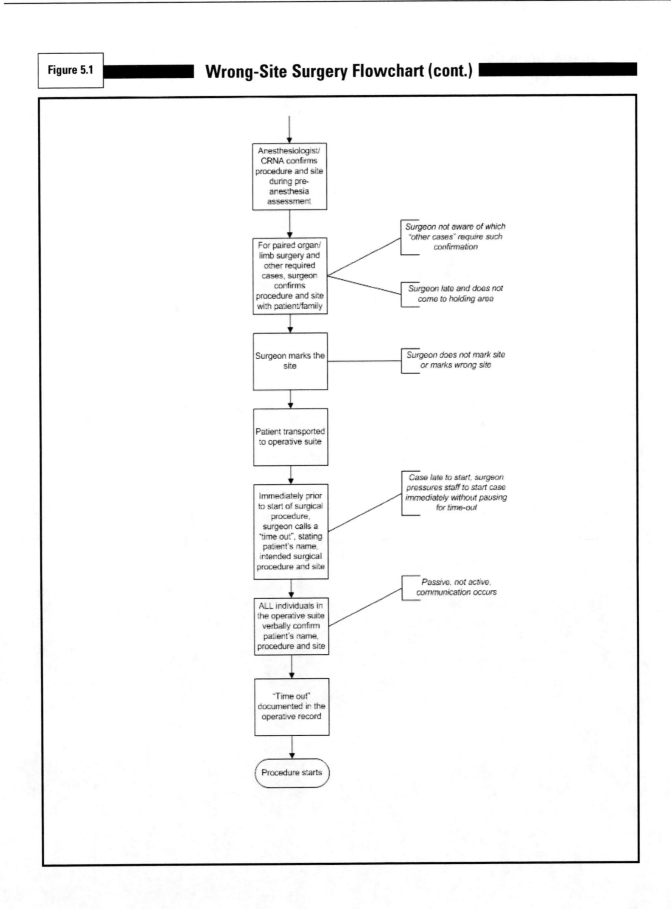

Figure 5.1   **Wrong-Site Surgery Flowchart (cont.)**

Step 3: Identify potential failure modes

The facilitator then led the FMEA team through a review of the finalized flowchart to identify individual steps in the process that might be vulnerable to break down. It included steps early on in the process (such as when the preadmission testing visit occurred) through to one of the final steps (when all individuals in the operative suite verbally confirm the patient's name, procedure, and site.)

The team added all the steps in the process to the flowchart (see Figure 5.1 for a sampling of these steps. For readability, not all of the failure modes that the FMEA team identified are affixed to the flowchart).

The potential failure modes were then entered into the matrix described in Chapter 1, and the group reached agreement on the frequency, severity, and detectability of the individual failure modes. From there, the team computed the risk priority number.

Step 4: Identify the potential effect of each failure mode

For each of the potential failure modes, the team identified the ultimate impact on the patient. For example, if the surgeon doesn't mark the site and no staff question this lapse, it's likely that wrong-site surgery will occur and the patient will be harmed. See Figure 5.2 for the completed FMEA matrix.

Figure 5.2 **Wrong-Site Surgery RPN**

Memorial Medical Center
Failure Modes and Effects Analysis
Privileged and Confidential

Process to be assessed: Wrong-site surgery

Potential failure mode	Potential effect of failure mode	Frequency (likeliness scale) 1–10	Severity (potential for harm) 1–10	Detectability (potential discovery) 1–10	Risk priority number
Surgeon's office staff posts wrong operative site	Surgical posting incorrect; confusion regarding correct site	2	10	10	200
Pre-admission testing call never occurs	Incorrect surgical posting not identified	1	4	2	8
Consent not completed/signed/accurate	Surgical site not documented or documented inaccurately	2	8	1	16
Patient sedated on floor, unable to participate in site verification process	Wrong procedure performed; incorrect patient or site	1	10	1	10
Patient incompetent, uncommunicative, or sedated; family not present operating room (OR) holding area	Wrong procedure performed; incorrect patient or site	2	10	1	10

Figure 5.2 ■ Wrong-Site Surgery RPN (cont.) ■

Potential failure mode	Potential effect of failure mode	Frequency (likeliness scale) 1–10	Severity (potential for harm) 1–10	Detectability (potential discovery) 1–10	Risk priority number
Consent form not in chart	Unable to confirm procedure or site	2	8	1	16
Surgeon not aware of which "other cases" require such confirmation	Procedures other than paired organs and limbs not verified or marked by surgeon	5	10	5	250
Surgeon late and does not come to holding area	Surgical site not marked prior to procedure	5	9	1	45
Patient is transported to OR suite with site unmarked	Surgical site not marked prior to procedure; greatly increases opportunity for wrong-site procedure	4	10	8	320
Surgeon does not mark site	Wrong-site procedure occurs	5	10	1	50
Surgeon does not mark site and no staff question this lapse	Wrong-site procedure occurs	8	10	7	560
Surgeon marks wrong site	Wrong-site procedure occurs	2	10	10	200
Case late to start, surgeon pressures staff to start case immediately without pausing for time-out	Wrong patient, procedure or surgical site occurs	6	10	3	180
Case late to start, surgeon pressures staff to start case immediately without pausing for time-out and case proceeds	Wrong patient, procedure or surgical site occurs	3	10	10	300
Passive, not active, communication occurs	Wrong patient, procedure or surgical site occurs	6	10	1	60

Step 5: Redesign the processes/underlying systems

The team's next step was to brainstorm potential improvements to the existing processes to reduce the risk of their breaking down and having the identified impact on the patient. For example, to reduce the risk of a failure of the surgeon to mark the site and staff questioning this lapse, the team developed the following strategies:

- The chief executive officer, chief of surgery, and OR clinical manager would drive cultural change in the OR so that nursing staff are comfortable addressing these issues with surgeon.

- Medical staff leadership and senior management would show clear, visible, and strong support of nursing staff in these efforts.

- Surgeons who don't follow the process will face medical staff disciplinary actions through the credentialing, privileging, and reappointment process.

For the complete results of this brainstorming session, see Figure 5.3.

Wrong-Site Surgery Risk-Reduction Efforts

Process to be assessed: **Pre-surgical process**

Potential failure mode	Responsible party	Risk priority number	Process improvement/risk reduction effort
Surgeon does not mark site and no staff question this lapse	Chief executive officer Chief of surgery Operating room clinical manager	560	Drive cultural change in the operating room (OR) whereby nursing staff are comfortable addressing these issues with surgeons. Medical staff leadership and senior management to show clear, visible, and strong support of nursing staff in these efforts. "Challenging" surgeons to be aggressively addressed through the medical staff disciplinary, credentialing, privileging, and reappointment process.
Patient is transported to OR suite with site unmarked	Supervisor, pre-operative holding	320	Implement the practice (with support of medical staff and senior management leadership) of not allowing any patient without a required site-marking to be transported from

Figure 5.3 **Wrong-Site Surgery Risk-Reduction Efforts (cont.)**

			pre-op holding to the OR suite (a "stop the line" strategy).
Case late to start, surgeon pressures staff to start case immediately without pausing for time-out and case proceeds.	OR clinical manager Chief of surgery	300	Implement the practice (with support of medical staff and senior management leadership) of not allowing any case to start without a time-out first being called (a "stop the line" strategy). Initiate a performance improvement effort aimed at reducing the incidence of cases starting late (eliminate the rush before the case).
Surgeon not aware of which "other cases" require such confirmation.	OR clinical manager Chief of surgery	250	Identify whether it is a knowledge deficit or issue of non-compliance (behavioral) and take appropriate action (education, monitoring, or counseling).
Surgeon's office staff posts wrong operative site.	Surgical case scheduler	200	(Although a relatively "less critical failure mode based upon its score, it was decided to address this issue due to its

Figure 5.3 **Wrong-Site Surgery Risk-Reduction Efforts (cont.)**

			high rating for "severity" and "detectability.") Implement a system whereby surgeons' office staff must have a double check/signoff of all surgical cases being scheduled (no verbal requests to schedule a case will be accepted unless followed up by a written/hard-copy request on the hospital-approved form).
Surgeon marks wrong site.		200	(Although a relatively "less critical failure mode" based upon its score, it was decided to address this issue due to its high rating for "severity" and "detectability.") Require documented evidence in the chart that the patient or family was involved in the marking process.

Step 6: Test and implement the redesigned process(es)

The team pilot-tested each of these risk-reduction strategies to determine the impact that such a change in process would have on the other processes within the surgical care process.

Step 7: Measure the effectiveness of the redesigned process

Step 8: Maintain the effectiveness of the redesigned process over time

The team carried out the wrong-site surgery FMEA final process improvements facility-wide and transitioned them into the organization's existing performance improvement process.

CHAPTER 5

RELATED ARTICLES

PROJECTS FOR IMPROVING SAFETY OF COUNTS IN THE OR

"What's so difficult about counting?" someone might think when he or she hears a sponge or instrument has been left in a patient. But counting in the operating room (OR) can be anything but simple. A single case may have hundreds of items. A deep cavity with a lot of blood can make it difficult to see. The OR can be noisy with multiple distractions.

In understanding an error-prone process, patient safety experts talk about human factors research, the study of the interaction between people and their environment. What is it about the environment that contributes to mistakes? Are there changes that could make the process safer?

A team at Stanford Hospital and Clinics in California is learning how complex counting is. It identified 20 potential "failure modes" in a sponge count before a case even began. The entire process from beginning to close had about 60 potential failure modes, notes Debra Gerardi, RN, MPH, JD, patient safety program manager at Stanford. "We need to look at all the variables, such as distraction and fatigue, that can set people up for failure," she says.

At M.D. Anderson Cancer Center in Houston, the OR staff, as part of a project on sponge counts, were asked to identify barriers that might affect accurate counts.

"We talked about how the perceived problems with sponge counts could create a slippery slope that leads to errors," says Judith Gerst, RN, MHA, CPHA, senior clinical quality analyst at M.D. Anderson and a former OR director.

Looking at failure modes

Stanford started its sponge count project in December as part of the Joint Commission on Accreditation of Healthcare Organizations' (JCAHO) requirement to analyze at least one high-risk process per year. A team of nine OR registered nurses (RNs), surgical technologists, a risk manager, and a quality manager has been meeting weekly with Gerardi as facilitator.

The team is doing an FMEA, a method borrowed from manufacturing and other industries for analyzing the safety risks in a process. The analysis involves breaking a process down into its steps, identifying where failures could occur, rating which of these failures would be the most serious, and planning improvements.

"We've been looking at the possible things that might go wrong at each step," says Gerardi. These might include the manufacturer sending an incomplete package of sponges, sponges not separated completely during the initial count, the count being interrupted, and different nurses and techs using slightly different methods to count. The next step will be to rate the risk of each failure mode and set priorities for process improvements. The Stanford team planned to begin implementing improvements this month.

What are the barriers?

As part of a performance improvement process at M.D. Anderson led by Sharon Land, RN, MBA, CNOR, director of perioperative services, Gerst introduced the staff to human factors. The staff then participated in a barrier analysis, asking, "What are the barriers to counting correctly?" Some factors identified included the following:

- Feeling rushed by surgeons and anesthesiologists
- Spending time socializing, then being hurried
- Not feeling comfortable speaking up
- Opening too many supplies so there was more to count
- No standard method of counting (staff who came from other hospitals used different methods)
- Nurses and techs not always counting together.

From these barriers, Gerst noted several "human factors" themes, such as

- A feeling of being "bulletproof" or "We can't make mistakes here. We are the best."

- An authority gradient: Nurses and techs were not willing to challenge physicians.

PROJECTS FOR IMPROVING SAFETY OF COUNTS IN THE OR (CONT.)

- Lack of teamwork: Someone might be angry with someone else and not feel inclined to cooperate.

Gerst and Land presented the findings to the staff as well as to the OR committee and surgeons in all of the sections. Meeting with the physicians, they told them the staff felt they were being rushed and were hesitant to challenge them. "We asked them, 'What are you going to do as surgeons to help this situation?'"

The department has also made a number of changes in count practices. The OR has been working on standardizing the counting process and educating staff on a uniform method.

For incorrect counts, a search is conducted of the field, the room, and the trash. No trash or linen is removed until the patient leaves the room. If the item is not found, the surgeon decides whether to take an x-ray. When counts are reported as correct, x-rays are not routinely done.

As a cancer facility, M.D. Anderson does not have many emergencies, which is a common indication for an x-ray. Regarding instruments, the policy is to take the following actions:

- An initial count on all cases

- A closing count by both the circulating nurse and scrub person on open peritoneum, abdominal, and thoracic cases

- A closing count by the scrub person on all other cases

- A count when the tray arrives in the reprocessing area

To monitor the process, Gerst tracks incident reports on incorrect counts. Results are reported to the OR committee and posted on the hospital's internal "dashboard," a collection of departmental statistics that is available electronically. The hospital as a whole has been working to strengthen its culture so issues related to errors are discussed more openly.

PROJECTS FOR IMPROVING SAFETY OF COUNTS IN THE OR (CONT.)

"We've been working to establish a nonpunitive, no-fear, no-blame environment," says Gerst. Part of that initiative is to develop a near-miss reporting system to encourage reporting of close calls so the organization can learn and work to prevent errors. Another part of the initiative focuses on developing a reward system for error and close-call reporting.

"People have to learn to trust this," says Gerst. "We also have been learning to get out of our silos, such as nursing and pharmacy, and learn from one another. All of this takes time to accept. We have been on this journey for three to five years."

Consistency of monitoring

At the University of Washington in Seattle, a multidisciplinary team with about 25 surgeons, anesthesia personnel, and nurses developed a quality improvement (QI) plan to reduce the potential for retained items. The major strategies are:

- Creating a position for a CQI nurse to keep the focus on patient safety. The nurse's role includes staff education, setting up indicators, monitoring, and giving the staff feedback about how they are doing. The nurse reports both to the director of surgical services and the director of quality improvement. "This is probably the most important step we have taken," says Judy Canfield, RNC, MNA, MBA, associate administrator of surgical services.

- Fully implementing counts for all cases with large open cavities on all services. A list of these cases was defined by a group of RNs and physicians. Among procedures on the list are abdominal and thoracic procedures, large urologic and gynecologic cases, and transplants. Not many orthopedic cases are included except hemipelvectomies.

- Refining instrument sets to reduce the number of items and make counting more efficient.

PROJECTS FOR IMPROVING SAFETY OF COUNTS IN THE OR (CONT.)

- Teaching and practicing how to count by all services.

- Monitoring the process to make sure counts are documented and are being done correctly. "It's the consistency of monitoring and feedback that helps keep us on track," says Canfield.

- For one year, performing an x-ray of 100% of the cases on the large-cavity list. The x-ray usually is taken in the postop area within 30 to 60 minutes of the end of the case. An initial reading is one by a resident or attending physician, with review by a radiologist within 24 hours. The CQI nurse monitors patient records for the readings.

As the QI project comes up on its one-year anniversary, "we'll review our CQI plan, as we have been through the year, for effectiveness, ease, and outcomes, then we'll go for the next steps, " says Canfield. One issue will be whether to continue x-rays for 100% of the large-cavity cases or to move to a different approach.

Source: "Projects for Improving Safety of Counts in the OR," OR Manager, March 2003. Reprinted with permission.

Chapter 6

CASE STUDY:
DELAY IN TREATMENT FMEA

CHAPTER 6

Case Study: Delay in Treatment FMEA

Another good example of an FMEA subject is delays in treatment. Approximately one-half of all sentinel events reviewed in the hospital emergency department (ED) setting were caused by delays in treatment, according to the Joint Commission on Accreditation of Healthcare Organization's (JCAHO) statistics on sentinel events. This issue rounds out the top five sentinel events the JCAHO has reviewed since 1995[1].

A JCAHO analysis in 2002 revealed that the ED was the most frequent care setting for sentinel events related to delays in treatment, followed closely by hospital intensive care units. The most common reasons reported for the delays in treatment include

- misdiagnosis
- delayed test results
- physician availability
- delayed administration of ordered care
- incomplete treatment
- delayed initial assessment
- patient left unattended

Like most of the other case studies presented in this book, sentinel events related to delays in treatment were most frequently caused by a breakdown in communication, most often with or

[1] *Sentinel event statistics, JCAHO Web site, www.jcaho.org, 2004.*

---

between physicians. Other common causes included shortcomings with the patient assessment process, discontinuity of care across settings or shifts, the orientation and training of staff, and availability of critical patient information.

This chapter will use the process outlined in Chapter 1 to present a case study of an FMEA on delay in treatment. This FMEA focuses on the management of the acute surgical patient who is admitted to the hospital in the middle of the night, as this scenario represents a high-risk, problem-prone process for many organizations. It is a process that involves a considerable coordination of effort between the ED physician, on-call surgeon, and nursing staff in the ED and on the inpatient unit. Given the significant number of hand-offs and the complex communication that must be executed, this topic makes an excellent target for an FMEA.

Step 1: Organize the team

The organization's leaders selected the following staff to participate in this process:

Core team members

- Chief operating officer
- Chief nurse executive
- Chief medical officer
- Risk manager, facilitator
- Clinical manager, intensive care unit
- Clinical manager, ED
- Charge nurse, medical/surgical unit
- Chief, emergency medicine
- Internist
- Intensivist
- Attending surgeon

Ad-hoc committee members

- Registered nurse, ED
- Licensed practical nurse, medical/surgical unit
- Two ED registered nurses
- Administrative director, radiology
- Administrative director, laboratory

Step 2: Flowchart the process

In a manner similar to the other case studies, using readily available software, the team flowcharted the medication use process, which appears in Figure 6.1 on the next two pages.

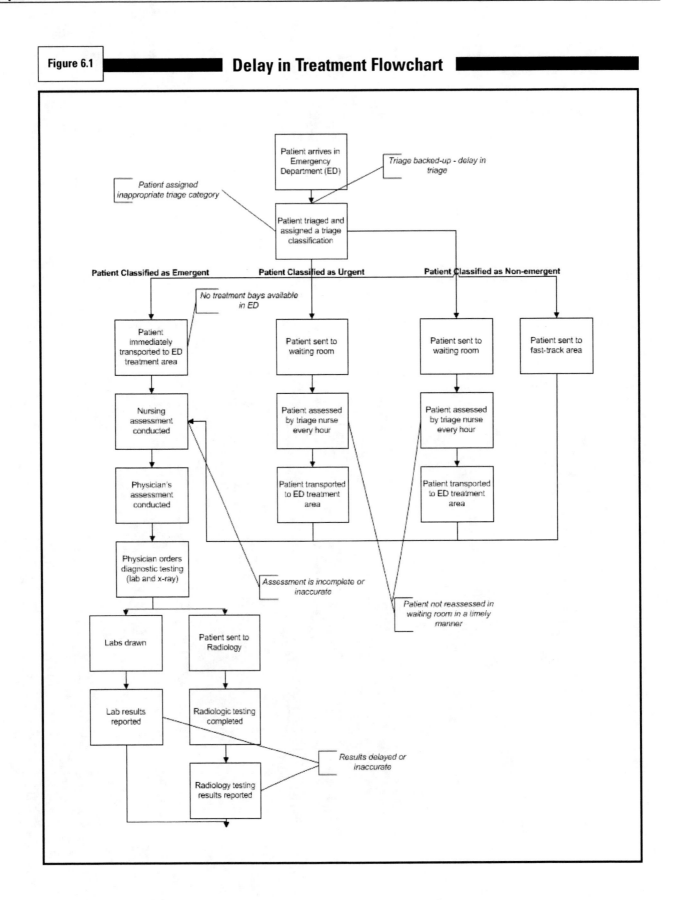

Figure 6.1 **Delay in Treatment Flowchart**

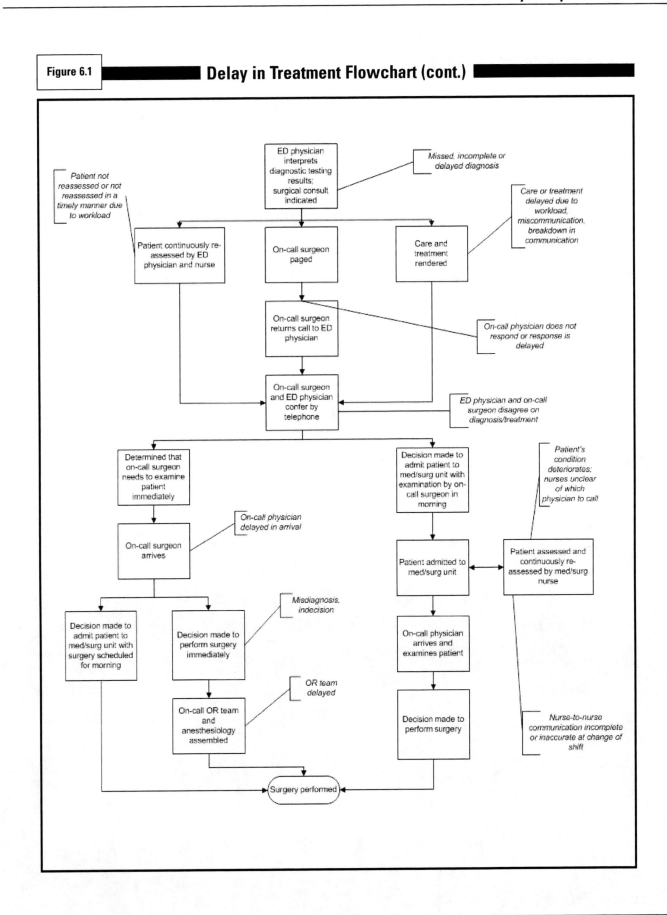

Figure 6.1 **Delay in Treatment Flowchart (cont.)**

Step 3: Identify potential failure modes

The facilitator then led the FMEA team through a review of the finalized flowchart to identify steps in the process that might be vulnerable to break down. For example, after a patient arrives in the ED, the hospital policy is for the patient to be triaged and assigned a triage classification. At this point in the process, two factors could cause the process to break down. The patient may be assigned an inappropriate category or triage may be backed up, causing a delay in triage. Other possible failure modes could occur at the point that lab or radiology testing results are reported. At that point, the results may be delayed or inaccurate. All potential failure modes were then added to the flowchart. See Figure 6.1 for a sampling of the areas identified.

The team then entered the potential failure modes into the matrix described in Chapter 1, and the group reached agreement on the frequency, severity, and detectability of the individual failure modes. From there, the team computed the risk priority numbers.

Step 4: Identify the potential effect of each failure mode

For each of the potential failure modes, the team identified the ultimate impact on the patient. For example, the team determined that a patient could be severely harmed (a score of 10, the highest possible score) if radiology or lab results were delayed because it could delay the initial diagnosis. Figure 6.2 reveals the results of the completed FMEA. Of special note is that 20 of the 21 identified failure modes give a score of 10 for potential of harm, even though the likeliness of the event occurring may be lower on the scale.

Figure 6.2

Delay in Treatment RPN

Process to be assessed: Delay in Treatment

Regional Medical Center
Failure Modes and Effects Analysis
Privileged and Confidential

Potential failure mode	Potential effect of failure mode	Frequency (Likeliness scale) 1–10	Severity (Potential for harm) 1–10	Detectability (Potential discovery) 1–10	Risk priority number
Triage backed-up	Delay in patient triage—patient's condition deteriorates	3	8	1	24
Patient assigned inappropriate triage category	Initial assessment and subsequent care not timely	1	10	10	100
No treatment bays available in emergency department (ED)	Delay in treatment	6	10	1	60
ED nursing assessment is incomplete or inaccurate	Inappropriate or delayed treatment	2	10	10	200
Patient not reassessed in waiting room in a timely manner	Patient's condition deteriorates without notice	5	10	7	350

Figure 6.2 — **Delay in Treatment RPN (cont.)**

Radiology or lab results delayed	Delay in initial diagnosis	7	10	4	280
Radiology or lab results inaccurate	Inaccurate diagnosis and subsequent treatment	2	10	10	200
Patient not assessed or not reassessed in ED in a timely manner due to workload	Patient's condition deteriorates without notice	5	10	5	250
Patient not reassessed in ED in a timely manner due to lack of staff diligence	Patient's condition deteriorates without notice	2	10	5	100
Missed, incomplete, or delayed diagnosis by ED physician	Patient condition deteriorates	2	10	10	200
Care or treatment delayed due to workload	Patient condition deteriorates	2	10	5	100
Care or treatment delayed due to miscommunication	Patient condition deteriorates	1	10	5	50
Care or treatment delayed due to lack of communication	Patient condition deteriorates	1	10	5	50
On-call physician does not respond to ED page or response is delayed	Delayed treatment	4	10	1	40
During telephone consultation between the	Delayed treatment;				

Figure 6.2   **Delay in Treatment RPN (cont.)**

ED physician and on-call surgeon, they disagree on diagnosis/treatment	Inappropriate treatment	3	10	9	270
On-call physician delayed in arriving to ED	Delayed diagnosis and treatment	4	10	1	40
Patient not reassessed or reassessed in a timely manner on medical/surgical unit	Patient condition deteriorates	3	10	10	300
Patient's condition deteriorates on medical/surgical unit; nurses unclear of which physician to call	Patient condition deteriorates	2	10	1	20
Misdiagnosis, indecision by surgeon	Delayed or inappropriate treatment	2	10	10	200
Medical/surgical unit nurse-to-nurse communication incomplete or inaccurate at change of shift	Ongoing care by nurse coming on shift is delayed or incorrect; critical status of patient is not known by nurse coming on shift	3	10	10	300
Operating room team delayed in arriving to hospital	Delay in critically needed surgery	1	10	1	10

Step 5: Redesign the processes/underlying systems

The next step was to brainstorm potential improvements to the existing processes to reduce the risk of their breaking down and having the identified impact on the patient. For example, to reduce the chance of a delay in the radiology or lab results, the team developed the following risk-reduction strategies, led by the administrative director of radiology:

- Have ED physicians interpret radiology files with over-reads by the radiologist.

- Subject radiology and the lab to a performance improvement study to measure, assess, and reduce test result turnaround time.

- Implement improvements as indicated.

To reduce the chance that a patient may not be reassessed in the waiting room in a timely manner, the team suggested the following risk-reduction strategies:

- Institute a standardized practice of reevaluating all patients in the ED waiting room once per hour. The ED charge nurse will conduct rounds on all patients and reassess their need for more timely care.

- The hospital will install a computerized patient-tracking system in the ED (triage room, fast-track area, and main ED treatment area) that identifies patients' time of arrival, triage category, current condition, and time that reassessment is due.

- The tracking system will provide the ability to monitor all patients for timely reassessment.

The full results of this session appear in Figure 6.3.

| Figure 6.3 | Delay in Treatment Risk-Reduction Efforts |

Memorial Medical Center

Failure Modes and Effects Analysis

Privileged and confidential

Process to be assessed: **Acute Surgical Admission Process**

Potential failure mode	Responsible party	Risk priority number	Process improvement/risk reduction effort
Patient not reassessed in waiting room in a timely manner	Clinical manager, emergency department chief, emergency medicine	350	Institute standardized practice of reevaluating all patients in emergency department (ED) waiting room once per hour. ED charge nurse will round on all patients and reassess their need for more timely care. A computerized patient tracking system will be installed in the ED (triage room, fast-track area, and main ED treatment areas) that identifies patient's time of arrival, triage category, current condition, time that reassessment is due, etc.). Tracking system will provide the ability to monitor all

---

Figure 6.3 ■ **Delay in Treatment Risk-Reduction Efforts (cont.)** ■

Failure	Responsible	RPN	Actions
Patient not reassessed or reassessed in a timely manner on medical/surgical unit	Charge nurse, medical/surgical unit Chief nurse executive	300	patients for timely reassessment. Reduce the patient load of charge nurses by one to two patients per shift to allow them sufficient time to review the (re)assessments conducted by the floor nurses. Revisit staffing plans and patterns on medical/surgical units, revising as necessary. Review standards for timeliness, completeness, and accuracy of assessments with nursing staff, assess their performance through 24-hour chart checks and take appropriate action (e.g., additional education, coaching or disciplinary action).
Med/surg unit nurse-to-nurse communication incomplete or inaccurate at change of shift	Charge nurse, medical/surgical unit Chief nurse executive	300	Revise the method of giving and receiving report between nurses at change of shift. Institute practice of walking rounds whereby the two nurses involved in the report of a given caseload walk from room to room, observing the patient and discussing the patient's condition and plan of care.
Radiology or lab results delayed	Administrative director, radiology	280	Institute practice of having ED physicians interpret radiology films with over-reads by radiologist. Subject radiology and lab to performance improvement study to measure, assess, and reduce test result turnaround

Figure 6.3 ▮▮▮ **Delay in Treatment Risk-Reduction Efforts (cont.)** ▮▮▮

	Chief, emergency medicine		time. Implement improvements as indicated.
	Chief, radiology		
During telephone consultation between the ED physician and on-call surgeon, they disagree on diagnosis/treatment	Chief, emergency medicine	270	Institute practice of requiring the on-call physician to come in to the ED and physically examine and assess patient if there is ever any disagreement on the patient's diagnosis or treatment.
	Chief, surgery		As part of the medical staff peer review process, the chiefs of emergency medicine, surgery, and internal medicine will review consultation cases weekly to assess the consistency between the ED and the on-call physicians' diagnosis and treatment decisions.
	Chief, internal Medicine		
Patient not reassessed or not reassessed in ED in a timely manner due to workload	Clinical manager, ED	250	Reassess staffing plans and patterns in ED, revising as necessary (especially staffing for peaks of activity and not averages).
	Charge nurse, ED		Revisit previous efforts to admit and physically transfer patients from ED to inpatient units in a timely manner.

Step 6: Test and implement the redesigned process(es)

The team then pilot-tested each of these risk-reduction strategies to determine the impact that such a change in process would have on the other processes within the system of the acute surgical admission process.

Step 7: Measure the effectiveness of the redesigned process

Step 8: Maintain the effectiveness of the redesigned process over time

The team carried out the final process improvements emanating from FMEA facility-wide and transitioned them into the organization's existing performance improvement process.

CHAPTER 6

RELATED ARTICLES

FOCUS ON EMERGENCY ROOM TREATMENT DELAYS: HOW STRESSED IS YOUR ED?

Emergency departments (EDs) are stretched to the seams, so much so that diversionary status, historically a seasonal occurrence, is now a year-round problem in many. And the flu season will soon be upon us! Now is the time to examine the contributing factors and potential risks particular to your hospital and to either implement new or retool current risk-reduction strategies.

Overcrowding

Overcrowding in EDs can be attributed to many factors. First, there is the seemingly ever-increasing number of patients seeking care due to:

- Increased utilization by uninsured individuals who lack access to other traditional medical services, such as urgent care facilities or private physician offices.

- Elder citizens on multiple medications and limited funds who frequently seek treatment in EDs to receive their maintenance medications to offset the costs of prescriptions not covered by Medicare in the ambulatory care setting.

- Recent legislation that has prompted less restrictive monitoring and benefits provided by health maintenance organizations (HMOs), resulting in increased utilization of EDs as urgent care facilities.

- The 24-hour availability of services.

But that doesn't tell the whole story. Overcrowding and delays are frequently attributable to system problems, not only within the ED but other hospital departments, as well. For example:

- Federal Emergency Medicine Treatment and Labor Act (EMTALA) legislation has created more demand on time and attention from ED staff, not only to screen, stabilize, and transfer patients, but also in documentation of the process.

- Inability to admit patients due to unavailability of inpatient beds.

FOCUS ON EMERGENCY ROOM TREATMENT DELAYS: HOW STRESSED IS YOUR ED? (CONT.)

- Slow reporting of diagnostic test results.

- Insufficient staffing.

- Slow response by specialty physicians.

- Ineffective communication.

Delay in treatment

The Joint Commission on Accreditation of Hospitals (JCAHO) recently issued a *Sentinel Event Alert* on delays in treatment in EDs. According to the Alert, EDs are the source of more than one-half of all reported sentinel event cases of patient death or permanent injury due to delays in treatment. The most commonly cited reason for a delay was misdiagnosis, followed by delayed test results, physician availability, delayed administration of treatment after being ordered, incomplete treatment, delayed initial assessment, patient left unattended, paging system malfunction, and inability to locate ED entrance.

Although risk managers may not be able to control the number of patients coming to the ED for care, they can take steps to control overcrowding and prevent a treatment delay sentinel event once they have arrived.

Consider implementing risk-reduction strategies to:

- Prevent overcrowding.

- Monitor diversionary status. Track and trend times and investigate contributing factors.

- Encourage physicians to discharge patients- both ED and inpatients—in a timely fashion.

FOCUS ON EMERGENCY ROOM TREATMENT DELAYS: HOW STRESSED IS YOUR ED? (CONT.)

Streamline patient flow and decrease the amount of time spent waiting for triage, medical screening exams, and treatment initiation by:

- Reviewing traffic patterns from admission to discharge.

- Identifying causes of logjams (e.g.. turnaround time for performing laboratory or radiology exams and reports).

- Implementing changes to promote efficient traffic flows, such as "fast track" or treatment protocols.

- Using concise, efficient documentation tools that limit documenting in multiple locations. (Consider using checklists.)

Ensure availability of specialty physicians

- Review and revise call lists and procedures for specialty physicians.

- Monitor response times and benchmark. Whenever possible maintain, a schedule of a First-call and a backup physician.

Provide adequate, competent staffing

- Review ED staffing patterns and plans.

- Staff for activity peaks, rather than averages.

- Evaluate staffing patterns in clinical support areas and adjust staffing patterns to include assigning diagnostic/clinical support staff dedicated to care of patients in the ED.

FOCUS ON EMERGENCY ROOM TREATMENT DELAYS: HOW STRESSED IS YOUR ED? (CONT.)

- Complete annual competency evaluations that include age-specific competencies, licensing, certifications, and credentialing.

- Conduct education and training on policies and procedures, clinical issues and patient safety for all staff, including float or agency staff.

Improve communication

- Engage in face-to-face transfer of care at shift change.

- Establish policies for follow-up communication on high-risk patients and for over-reads on diagnostic test results. This should include a recall or tickler system.

- Implement policies prohibiting telephone advice by non-physicians.

- Maintain a system to document all telephone calls (even if the only information or instruction given is to "come to the ED").

- Keep a current list of translators.

- Provide patients with written discharge instructions.

- Document all consultations with specialists or attending physicians.

- Reduce the practice of verbal orders; however, when necessary, make it a practice to read back all verbal orders.

A high volume of patients seeking care, coupled with staffing shortages, increased patient acuity, breakdown in communication, and a lack of knowledge, skills, or resources that promote quality patient care increase risk exposures in the ED. It is advisable to review your programs now, before the cold winter months blow in, bringing with them an increased patient volume to your already stressed ED.

Reprinted with permission from STATHealth Care Newsletter, Chubb, Warren, NJ.

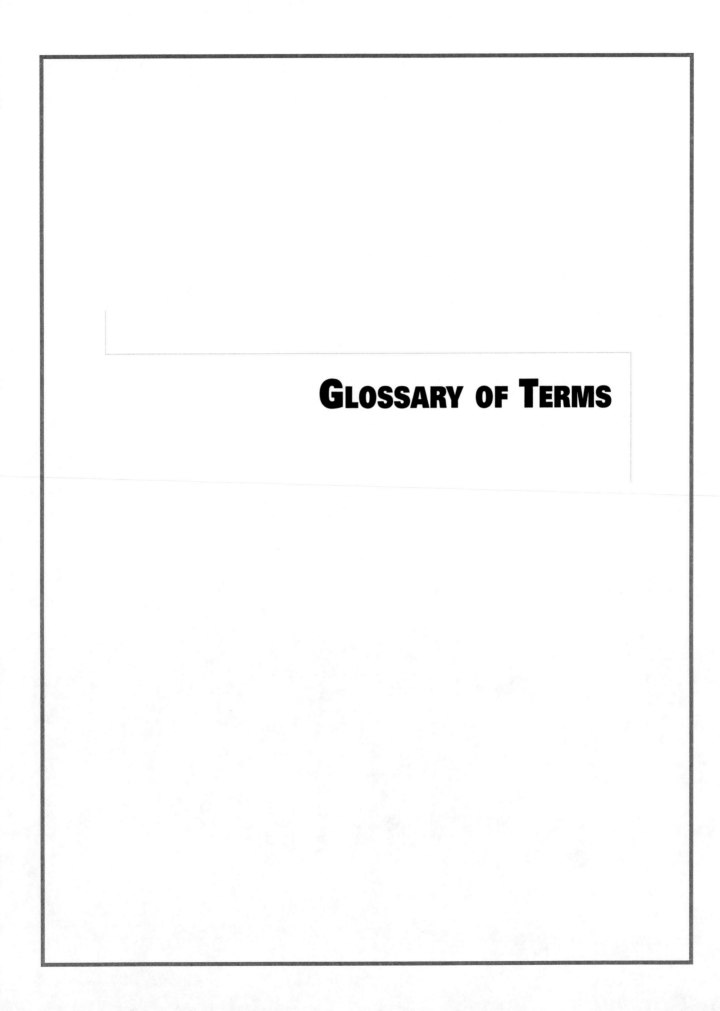

GLOSSARY OF TERMS

Glossary of Terms

This glossary contains definitions of many terms related to Failure Modes and Effects Analysis that are used throughout this book.

Common cause: A statement of a condition that is responsible for many past events.

Detectability: How easily the failure is recognized or discovered.

Effects: The possible outcomes that a breakdown or failure could have on patients and the seriousness of those possible outcomes.

Face validity: A quick assessment to determine if something makes sense or if it appears to be well-grounded on the surface.

Facilitator: Someone who is knowledgeable of and well versed in the process of conducting a Failure Modes and Effects Analysis. The facilitator should also be nonjudgmental, encourage all of the team members to participate and share their insight, and keep the discussion going.

Failure modes: Identifies the ways the process could break down or fail.

Failure Modes and Effects Analysis (FMEA): A powerful, systematic, and analytic tool used to identify where people, equipment, supplies, information, systems, and processes can "go wrong" or malfunction—and prevent them from doing so. FMEAs are also used to reduce the impact of the malfunction on the process, system, person, or other ultimate outcome.

Frequency: How likely it is for the failure to occur.

Hard-wired actions: Forcing functions, such as installing engineering controls (e.g., lock-out functions on endoscopy decontamination equipment or barcoding labels on blood products), automation, and computerization.

Hazard vulnerability assessment: The identification of potential emergencies and the direct and indirect effects these emergencies may have on the health care organization's operations and the demand for its services.

High-risk process: Processes that if not carried out correctly, have a significant potential for affecting the safety of the patient.

Joint Commission on Accreditation of Healthcare Organizations (JCAHO): An independent, non-profit organization, which is the primary accreditor of health care organizations in the United States. It evaluates and accredits nearly 17,000 health care organizations—including hospitals, nursing homes, health care networks, managed care organizations, home care organizations, mental health organizations, ambulatory care centers, assisted living facilities, and clinical laboratories. It lists its standards in the *Comprehensive Accreditation Manual for Hospitals*. The JCAHO surveys organizations on actual performance—rather than the capability to perform—as well as the quality of their plans or policies and how well different departments and disciplines work together to perform improvements.

Medication error: The National Coordinating Council for Medication Error Reporting and Prevention defines a medication error as "any preventable event that may cause or lead to inappropriate medication use or patient harm while the medication is in the control of the health care professional, patient, or consumer. Such events may be related to professional practice, health care products, procedures or systems, including prescribing; order communication; product labeling, packaging, and nomenclature; compounding; dispensing; distribution; administration; education; monitoring; and use."

Near-misses (also called close calls): An incident or process variation that doesn't effect a patient's outcome, but if it reoccurred could cause a serious adverse event. Near-misses are events that fall under the JCAHO's Sentinel Event policy. (See definition for sentinel event.)

Performance improvement: The continuous monitoring, analyzing, and improving of all processes in a health care organization that directly or indirectly affect patient care. Performance improvement is one of the most important functions a health care organization can accomplish, according to the JCAHO.

Risk priority number (RPN): The frequency multiplied by the severity multiplied by the detectability.

Root cause analysis: An in-depth investigation to determine why a sentinel event occurred.

Sentinel event: The JCAHO defines a sentinel event as an "unexpected occurrence involving death or serious physical or psychological injury, or the risk thereof." The JCAHO requires health care organizations to undergo a root cause analysis or "intensively" analyze sentinel events and other "undesirable patters or trends in performance," and to take action to "reduce the risk of sentinel events." It also requires hospital leaders to define and carry out the processes for identifying and managing sentinel events.

Severity: How serious the impact of this failure is on the patient.

Transfusion error: A complication of blood transfusion where there is an immune response against the transfused blood cells or other components of the transfusion.

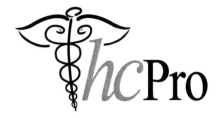

Related Products from HCPro

Maximize Patient Safety with Advanced Root Cause Analysis

For years, the JCAHO's leadership and performance improvement standards have required root cause analysis, but hospitals tend to fall short of finding the true causes of problems. This book will explain to readers how to break through those barriers and use six steps to identify the underlying cause of a medical error or system failure. Specifically, it

- explains in easy-to-understand language the problems associated with a root cause analysis and what you can do to avoid them
- offers examples, case studies, and best-practice advice on root cause and common cause analysis
- provides expert advice from the partners of Performance Improvement International, a distinguished leader in error reduction

Performance Improvement: Winning Strategies for Quality and JCAHO Compliance, Third Edition—Plus CD/ROM

This is the third edition of our award-winning compliance tool! The book and companion CD/ROM have just been updated to reflect the significant changes in the JCAHO's survey process. The JCAHO has revamped its PI standards—specifically around ORYX, FMEA, and core measures—and made PI one of the only remaining planned interviews in the 2004 survey process. You need to know how to respond to the changes to comply! Plus—in addition to keeping PI and quality of care a main focus of its survey process, the JCAHO is adding patient safety as a critical area as well. This book includes a new chapter on patient safety in response to the JCAHO's increased focus on this crucial area, and an educational PowerPoint presentation on CD/ROM.

JCAHO 2003 and 2004 National Patient Safety Goals: Successful Strategies for Compliance

Hospitals continue to struggle to meet the intent of the JCAHO's National Patient Safety Goals. This step-by-step tool breaks down each of the requirements within the JCAHO's seven National Patient Safety Goals and provides you with a series of best-practice tips that you can easily implement. You'll receive

- CASE STUDIES from hospitals across the country that are successfully complying with these seven Goals
- sample POLICIES, including patient identification and verification of operative site policies

---

- step-by-step ADVICE, such as how to prevent wrong-site/ patient/procedure surgery
- sample FORMS and CHECKLISTS, including a surgery verification checklist

Preparing Your Patient Safety Program for JCAHO Survey

Your patient safety program initiatives have never been under more scrutiny than right now. From the JCAHO's new Patient Safety Goals to new survey expectations, you need to make sure your patient safety program is up to par. This book provides you with

- plain-English EXPLANATIONS of the JCAHO's 2004 patient safety standards and step-by-step ADVICE on how to comply with them
- sample CHECKLISTS, FORMS, and DOCUMENTS
- INSIGHT into how your patient safety initiatives will be surveyed
- TIPS and GUIDANCE on implementing a patient safety program, failure modes and effects analysis (FMEA), sentinel events, and root cause analysis
- EXAMPLES of the types of patient safety questions surveyors might ask staff

Newsletters

Briefings on JCAHO

This 12-page monthly newsletter is the respected voice of authority for practical, independent guidance on succeeding in the accreditation process at thousands of hospitals nationwide. It will keep you up to speed on all JCAHO changes and provide invaluable insight into how the new JCAHO survey process unfolds. Whether readers are new to the survey game or seasoned professionals, each newsletter offers quick reading "how-to" advice on meeting the JCAHO standards. You'll receive tips and information from accreditation experts that would otherwise cost you dearly in consulting fees and research!

Briefings on Patient Safety

From medication management to the Patient Safety Goals, there has never been more focus on your facility's patient safety initiatives than right now. This monthly resource was created exclusively to help you provide a safe environment of care for your patients. From best-practice information regarding medication management to ensuring that your patient safety program stands up to JCAHO scrutiny, you'll have the tools you need to succeed!

To obtain additional information, to order any of the above products, or to comment on *Failure Modes and Effects Analysis: Building Safety Into Everyday Practice,* please contact us at:

Mail:	**Toll-free telephone:** 800/650-6787
HCPro	**Toll-free fax:** 800/639-8511
P.O. Box 1168	**E-mail:** *customerservice@hcpro.com*
Marblehead, MA 01945	**Internet:** *www.hcpro.com*
